Human remains
and mass violence

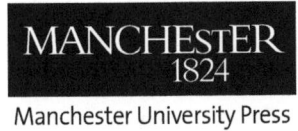
Manchester University Press

HUMAN REMAINS AND VIOLENCE

Human remains and violence aims to question the social legacy of mass violence by studying how different societies have coped with the dead bodies resulting from war, genocide and state-sponsored brutality. However, rather paradoxically, given the large volume of work devoted to the body on the one hand, and to mass violence on the other, the question of the body in the context of mass violence remains a largely unexplored area and even an academic blind spot. Interdisciplinary in nature, *Human remains and violence* intends to show how various social and cultural treatments of the dead body simultaneously challenge common representations, legal practices and morality. This series aims to provide proper intellectual and theoretical tools for a better understanding of mass violence's aftermaths.

Series editors

Jean-Marc Dreyfus & Élisabeth Anstett

Also available in this series

Destruction and human remains: disposal and concealment in genocide and mass violence
Edited by Élisabeth Anstett & Jean-Marc Dreyfus

Governing the dead: sovereignty and the politics of dead bodies
Edited by Finn Stepputat

Human remains and mass violence

Methodological approaches

Edited by

Jean-Marc Dreyfus & Élisabeth Anstett

Manchester University Press

Copyright © Manchester University Press 2015

While copyright in the volume as a whole is vested in Manchester University Press, copyright in individual chapters belongs to their respective authors, and no chapter may be reproduced wholly or in part without the express permission in writing of both author and publisher.

Published by Manchester University Press
Altrincham Street, Manchester M1 7JA, UK
www.manchesteruniversitypress.co.uk

British Library Cataloguing-in-Publication Data is available

ISBN 978 1 5261 1674 1 *paperback*
ISBN 978 0 7190 9650 1 *hardback*

First published by Manchester University Press in hardback 2015

This edition first published 2017

The publisher has no responsibility for the persistence or accuracy of URLs for any external or third-party internet websites referred to in this book, and does not guarantee that any content on such websites is, or will remain, accurate or appropriate.

Printed by Lightning Source

Contents

List of contributors   *page* vii

Acknowledgements   xi

    Introduction. Corpses and mass violence: an inventory of the unthinkable   1
    Élisabeth Anstett & Jean-Marc Dreyfus

1 The biopolitics of corpses of mass violence and genocide   12
    Yehonatan Alsheh

2 Seeking the dead among the living: embodying the disappeared of the Argentinian dictatorship through law   44
    Sévane Garibian

3 The human body: victim, witness and evidence of mass violence   56
    Caroline Fournet

4 Moral discourse and action in relation to the corpse: integrative concepts for a criminology of mass violence   81
    Jon Shute

5 The disposal of corpses in an ethnicized civil war: Croatia, 1941–45   106
    Alexander Korb

6 Renationalizing bodies? The French search mission for
   the corpses of deportees in Germany, 1946–58   129
   Jean-Marc Dreyfus

7 From bones-as-evidence to tutelary spirits: the status of
   bodies in the aftermath of the Khmer Rouge genocide   146
   Anne Yvonne Guillou

8 Display, concealment and 'culture': the disposal of bodies
   in the 1994 Rwandan genocide   161
   Nigel Eltringham

9 An anthropological approach to human remains from
   the gulags   181
   Élisabeth Anstett

Index   199

Contributors

Yehonatan Alsheh wrote his doctoral dissertation in the Tel Aviv University School of Historical Studies on the political and intellectual origins of the United Nations Genocide Convention. He developed with Professor Yair Auron an Open University undergraduate programme on comparative genocide studies, consisting of 12 textbooks, and the first programme of its kind to appear in Hebrew and to be taught in Israeli academia. So far almost 5,000 students have been on the course, including around 200 Palestinian political prisoners. He is currently a Postdoctoral Fellow at the Balsillie School of International Affairs, Wilfrid Laurier University, Ontario, Canada. He has published in Hebrew, English, Spanish and Afrikaans.

Élisabeth Anstett has been a social anthropologist and tenured research scholar at the Centre National de la Recherche Scientifique (CNRS) in Paris since October 2009, and is a member of IRIS (Interdisciplinary Research Institute on Social issues). Her area of expertise covers Europe and the post-socialist world, on which she has published extensively. Her recent works focus on the way post-Soviet societies are dealing with the traces left by the Soviet concentration camp system, among which are mass graves, and more broadly on the legacies of mass violence in eastern Europe, especially in Russia and Belarus. She has published, among other works, *Une Atlantide russe: anthropologie de la mémoire en Russie* *postsoviétique* (La Découverte, 2007) and co-edited with Luba Jurgenson *Le Goulag en héritage, pour une anthropologie de la trace* (Pétra, 2009).

Jean-Marc Dreyfus is Reader in Holocaust Studies within the Department of History at the University of Manchester. His research interests include: Holocaust studies; genocide studies and the anthropology of genocide; the history of the Jews in Europe in the nineteenth and twentieth centuries, especially in France; the economic history of France and Germany; Holocaust memory and the politics of memory; the modern history of Alsace; and the rebuilding of post-war societies. He is the author of four monographs, including *Pillages sur ordonnances: la confiscation des banques juives en France et leur restitution, 1940–1953* (Fayard, 2003); with Sarah Gensburger, *Nazi Labour Camps in Paris* (Berghahn Books, 2012); and *Il m'appelait Pikolo: un compagnon de Primo Levi raconte* (*He Called Me Pikolo: A Companion of Primo Levi Tells His Story*) (Robert Laffont, 2007). He is the co-editor of the *Dictionnaire de la Shoah* (*Dictionary of the Holocaust*) (Larousse, 2009).

Nigel Eltringham teaches social anthropology at the University of Sussex. He has published extensively on the aftermath of the 1994 Rwandan genocide, and has conducted research in Rwanda, among the Rwandan diaspora in Europe and at the International Criminal Tribunal for Rwanda (Arusha Tanzania). He is the author of *Accounting for Horror: Post-Genocide Debates in Rwanda* (Pluto, 2004), editor of *Framing Africa: Portrayals of a Continent in Contemporary Mainstream Cinema* (Berghahn, 2013) and co-editor, with Pam Maclean, of *Remembering Genocide* (Routledge, 2014).

Caroline Fournet is Associate Professor and Rosalind Franklin Fellow at the Department of Criminal Law and Criminology at the University of Groningen. She was previously Senior Lecturer at Exeter University's School of Law. Her main publications include three monographs: *International Crimes: Theories, Practice and Evolution*, with an Introduction by Professor Malcolm N. Shaw QC (Cameron, 2006); *The Crime of Destruction and the Law of Genocide: Their Impact on Collective Memory* (Ashgate, 2007); and *Genocide and Crimes Against Humanity: Confusions and Amalgams in French Practice* (Hart Publishing, 2013), which was awarded a British Academy Small Research Grant for its completion. Her current research includes several comparative works on international criminal law and justice as well as on human rights law. She is also a co-investigator on the ERC-funded research programme Corpses of Mass Violence and Genocide and the Editor for Law for the academic journal *Human Remains and Violence: An Interdisciplinary Journal*.

Sévane Garibian is Doctor of Law from the Universities of Paris X and Geneva, Assistant Professor at the University of Geneva (Grantholder of Excellence UNIGE 2011) and Lecturer at the University of Neuchâtel, Switzerland, where she teaches legal philosophy and international criminal law. Her work focuses on law relating to mass crimes (international criminal justice, transitional justice, human rights, memory laws). She has been a Swiss National Science Foundation Postdoctoral Research Fellow (2008–12) and a Visiting Fellow at the University of Buenos Aires (2008–12) and at the University Pompeu Fabra of Barcelona (since 2012). She is currently working on the legal treatment of the dictatorial past in Argentina and Spain, with a monograph in preparation. She is the author of numerous papers and contributions to anthologies, as well as two books, *Le Crime contre l'humanité au regard des principes fondateurs de l'Etat moderne: Naissance et consécration d'un concept* (Schulthess, LGDJ, Bruylant, 2009) and, with co-author Alberto Puppo, *Normas, valores, poderes: Ensayos sobre Positivismo y Derecho internacional* (Fontamara, Doctrina Jurídica, 2010).

Anne Yvonne Guillou is Doctor in Anthropology at the École des Hautes Études en Sciences Sociales (Institute of Higher Studies in Social Sciences), Paris. She holds a BA in Khmer language and culture from the Institut National des Langues et Civilisations orientales (National Institute of Asian Languages and Civilizations), Paris. As a tenured researcher at the Centre National de la Recherche Scientifique (CNRS, French National Centre of Scientific Research), she is currently working in the Centre Asie du Sud-Est (CASE, Centre of Southeast Asian Studies), Paris. Her current research interests are in social suffering and post-genocide social and ritual recovery; and Khmer popular religious systems. She is the author of the book *Cambodge, soigner dans les fracas de l'histoire: médecins et société* (Les Indes Savantes, 2009) and has co-edited a multi-author volume as a guest editor (with S. Vignato), *Life After Collective Death in Southeast Asia* (a two-part special issue of *Southeast Asia Research*, published by the School of Oriental and African Studies, University of London, 2012, 2013).

Alexander Korb is Lecturer in Modern European History at the University of Leicester and deputy director of the Stanley Burton Centre for Holocaust and Genocide Studies, UK. He is the author of numerous articles about the Holocaust and war and genocide in south-eastern Europe. With his last book, *Im Schatten des Weltkriegs: Massengewalt der Ustaša gegen Serben, Juden und Roma in Kroatien 1941–1945* (Hamburger Edition, 2013) he won the Fraenkel Prize in Contemporary History and numerous other awards. In his current project he explores how German journalists wrote about Europe between the 1920s and the 1970s.

Jon Shute is a criminologist working in the Centre for Criminology and Criminal Justice (CCCJ) in the School of Law at the University of Manchester. With a background in psychology, he has enduring research interests in human development, family stress and, more recently, the criminology of mass violence. He is a co-investigator on the ERC-funded research programme Corpses of Mass Violence and Genocide and a member of the European Society of Criminology's Atrocity Crime and Transitional Justice Working Group. He is also part of the 'Eurogang' international network of gang researchers. He teaches and supervises in the areas of psychological criminology and the criminology of mass violence.

Acknowledgements

It was with the help of numerous research institutions that we were able to organize the workshop held in Paris on 23–24 June 2011 that led to the creation of this book. We would therefore like to warmly thank, for their crucial financial support, the Centre d'histoire de Sciences-Po in Paris (for the venue); Jeremy Gregory and James Thompson at the School of Arts, Languages and Cultures, University of Manchester; Dominique Memmi at la Maison des Sciences de l'Homme Paris-Nord; and the Institut de Recherche Interdisciplinaire sur les Enjeux Sociaux (Paris), as well as its directors, Didier Fassin and Marc Bessin. Additionally, Estelle Girard (CNRS-IRIS, Paris) and the team at IRIS must be thanked for organizing the workshop.

We are also grateful to the following people for their enthusiastic participation at the Paris workshop: Elisabeth Claverie (CNRS, Paris, France), Alexandra Onfray (magistrate, France), Richard Rechtman (EHESS, Paris, France), Michael Salter (University of Central Lancashire, UK), Jacques Sémelin (CERI, Sciences-Po, Paris, France), Michel Signoli (CNRS, Marseille, France), Finn Stepputat (DIIS, Denmark), Marc Taccoen (Institut Medico-Légal, Paris, France), Bertrand Taithe (University of Manchester, UK) and Sari Wastell (Goldsmith College, UK). Their ongoing commitment to our topic was essential to the open and engaging dialogue at the workshop, and to the rigour that was carried through to this volume.

Finally, we would like to thank the European Research Council for supporting both the publication of this volume and the wider research environment from which it has arisen.

Élisabeth Anstett & Jean-Marc Dreyfus

Introduction. Corpses and mass violence: an inventory of the unthinkable

Élisabeth Anstett & Jean-Marc Dreyfus

Mass violence is one of the defining phenomena of the twentieth century, which some have even called the 'century of genocides'.[1] Scarred by the Armenian genocide, the *Holodomor* in Ukraine, the Spanish Civil War, the Holocaust, the gulags and, more recently, the crimes against humanity committed in Bosnia, Europe alone offers a range of examples of such extreme events.[2] These outbreaks of mass violence particularly affected civilians, unlike most previous massacres, with the motivations behind them political, ideological, racial or religious, and fitted into a generalized background of violence and the construction of nation-states or territorial empires.[3] Mass violence was also a symptom of new types of political regime, with no precedent in human history.[4] Yet, in spite of their scale and variety, and in spite of their millions of victims, European massacres and genocides on their own do not allow us to draw a definitive typology of mass violence, for other continents have seen, and indeed are still witnessing, massacres which continually widen our notions of these human catastrophes.

Asia, for instance, has been scarred not only by the Great Chinese Famine, which, according to some estimates, claimed up to 40 million victims during the policy of the 'Great Leap Forward',[5] but also by the Cambodian genocide, which resulted in 1.5 million deaths between 1975 and 1979,[6] along with the mass violence committed in Indonesia under the Suharto regime, which has to be considered in terms of both its political and its ethnic character.[7]

Africa has suffered the Rwandan genocide, which claimed 800,000 victims over the course of just three months in 1994,[8] and the sporadic yet recurring violence in Sudan since 1982, which has claimed over 2 million victims in total, many of them in Darfur,[9] while specialists in this field find it difficult even to agree on what to call the constantly mutating cycle of violence which has claimed 4 million victims since 1994 in the Democratic Republic of Congo (formerly Zaire), and which has become far more than a simple aftershock from the Rwandan genocide. The continent of America has seen political 'disappearances' under Argentina's military dictatorship,[10] along with mass killings in Guatemala between 1981 and 1983,[11] and the successive waves of violence which have shaken Haiti since the beginning of the twentieth century. Taken together, these further genocides and massacres force us to consider the European experience in light of mass violence perpetrated across the globe throughout the twentieth century.

The social sciences, although somewhat slow to address the phenomenon of genocide, have recently brought a variety of new perspectives to the questions it poses. Academic studies of mass violence have a rather complex history, closely linked to general developments in the human sciences as well as the political contexts within which the research has been carried out. These studies have been strongly structured around the questions raised by the Holocaust, which they have placed in a wider comparative context in an attempt to define certain anthropological fundamentals and, where possible, constants. Along with comparative studies of mass violence,[12] a growing number of monographs[13] have brought into focus the fact that while it has been possible to study some genocides soon after the event, other instances of mass violence have had to wait for a favourable political context to emerge, along with freer access to archives, before they could be documented. These studies draw on the approaches of such varied disciplines as law, history, political science and anthropology, and focus on questions as wide-ranging as the mechanisms of decision,[14] the definition of victims,[15] transitional justice[16] and the memory of mass violence.[17] Important contributions from the fields of law,[18] history[19] and anthropology[20] have together led to the establishment of a new disciplinary field, that of genocide studies, which has been consolidated through the creation of collaborative networks (the International Network of Genocide Scholars in Europe and the International Association of Genocide Scholars in the USA), academic publications (the journals *Holocaust and Genocide*

Studies, Journal of Genocide Research and *Genocide Studies and Prevention*) and annual conferences.

In spite of the large amount of work produced so far within this field – paradoxically even, given the importance of the body as a topic in the social sciences – the question of the body in relation to mass violence remains a largely unexplored theme. Over the last thirty years, studies centred on the body have evolved considerably, thanks to the growing importance in the English-speaking world of cultural studies, with its innovative view of the body as the meeting point of diverse social and cultural forces. This vision of the body as not only a resonant marker of identity on many levels, but also as the ultimate seat of affect, provides a solid starting point for a reading of human cultures as a coherent whole, whether as part of a literary, or biological or historical approach. The body, then, is a theme which not only runs across all the human sciences,[21] but also possesses longstanding legitimacy and has recently seen an upsurge in interest in light of technological developments and the emergence of the concept of biopower.[22]

Yet, while the body, when alive, is considered from almost every possible perspective by the social sciences, it has so far been paid virtually no attention once dead. Only archaeologists and anthropologists have sought to provide an account of the religious and political significance with which it is invested in various contexts.[23] Yet human remains constitute a grey area, or even a taboo, in the research on the body conducted in the human sciences. Studies on the subject are few[24] and virtually no work has been done on the presence of the body at the scenes of mass crime (with the exception of that done by Becker[25]). Yet the fate of the body, and more particularly that of the corpse, in our view constitutes a fundamental key to understanding genocidal processes and the impact of mass violence on contemporary societies.

The study of how the dead body is treated can lead us to an understanding of the impact of mass violence on contemporary societies – from the moment of the infliction of death until the stage when the bodies of the victims are reinstated in a peaceful society. This belief has encouraged us to put in place a vast research programme, entitled 'Corpses of Mass Violence and Genocide', financed by a grant from the European Research Council (ERC) from July 2011.[26] To address the issue of the practical and symbolic treatment of corpses by societies affected by mass violence, we proposed to maintain a qualitative, comparative and multidisciplinary approach. The qualitative dimension enables us to draw support from the documented analysis of a range of studies, each examining specific historical and cultural scenarios. These cases are, however, potentially so numerous that it seemed to us imperative at the start to limit ourselves to the contemporary period. Starting from research on mass violence in Europe (the Holocaust for Jean-Marc Dreyfus and the gulag for Élisabeth Anstett), it seemed to us necessary to engage in a comparative dialogue with specialists on mass crimes perpetrated elsewhere in the world, such as Rwanda,[27] Cambodia[28] and Argentina.[29] Moreover, in the knowledge that an approach within a single discipline would be insufficient to bring out all the issues pertaining to the fate of the corpses resulting from mass violence, and in light of the latter's complexity, we have decided upon a multidisciplinary approach. This involves a close dialogue between anthropology – whether social[30] or medico-legal[31] – within the domain of violence and the following disciplines: history, which reconstructs the time and place of the atrocities;[32] law, which was the first discipline to be engaged in a systemic analysis of mass crimes and to have endeavoured to establish a theoretical framework;[33] and political science, from the founding works of Hannah Arendt,[34] which brought some structure to the field, up to the studies conducted by Pierre Hassner[35] and Jacques Sémelin[36] on the genesis of extreme violence.

Anticipating the epistemological, methodological and ethical issues raised by our intellectual project, we held a two-day workshop in June 2011 to enable our team to draw an inventory of the conceptual and methodological tools available for addressing the corpse in mass violence, and thus to establish a panorama of ideas and approaches available to address the dead body in genocide scenarios. We had also to ask ourselves about the possibility of addressing these seemingly impossible aspects of the subject of corpses en masse, as well as working on the definition of a vocabulary – if not a grammar – of shared research. The result of this collective thinking both provides an inventory of the terms of art in our various disciplines and throws light on current conundrums and the genuine difficulties in grasping an extreme, but in our view essential, topic.

Therefore the contributions collected here address matters as diverse and crucial as the definition of our aims, the specificity of our methods and our respective ethical standpoints. To probe the intellectual framework existing today for the recognition of the object 'body/corpse', we invited the political scientist Yehonatan Alsheh to examine the concept of biopower, in chapter 1. This theory – developed by Michel Foucault – has in effect become the most commonly used tool of reference in the social and political sciences when it is necessary to address the relationships of power exerted on bodies and to study the punitive or disciplinary procedures deployed by states. In this seminal chapter, Alsheh shows the undeniable contribution and the limits of the biopower theory in the understanding of dead bodies en masse.

While the corpse continues to be a body, it is no less true that this singular object changes its status with its own change of state, and all the more readily so if it is found to be broken, denatured or destroyed (in whole or in part). Hence, it seemed to us essential to clarify the definition of these objects, the status (symbolic as well as juridical) that is accorded to them in our fields and the functions specifically assigned to them. The jurists Sévane Garibian and Caroline Fournet have tackled this task in chapters 2 and 3. The former is concerned with the possibility that law allows to embody the disappeared and the latter with the place international criminal law gives to the body. The criminologist Jon Shute in chapter 4 ponders the fact that criminology – the science of crime – has for so long ignored mass crime, even though the link between the corpse and the criminal is one of the fundamentals of the discipline. Alex Korb for his part has chosen a different approach in chapter 5, largely drawing on German archives to describe the various modalities of treatment of corpses in occupied Croatia, a country from 1941 a satellite state of the Reich and the theatre of particularly murderous inter-ethnic conflicts. He shows how working ideologies along with historical legacy and geographical landscapes determined the disposal of the bodies. As an extension to the criminological approach, the historian Jean-Marc Dreyfus examines in chapter 6 the simultaneously diplomatic and medico-legal nature of the activities of the French Search Commission for Corpses of Deportees in Germany. In its quest for the identification of the remains of French deportees throughout the territory of the former Reich, the Commission exhumed and identified thousands of corpses between 1946 and 1957, bringing a fund of unprecedented expertise into the areas of diplomacy and science.

It falls to the anthropologist to clarify in the final and frank analyses the ethical and epistemological difficulties that give rise to these singular objects of corpses en masse. The impacts for researchers and societies are considered: in Cambodia by Anne Yvonne Guillou (chapter 7), in Rwanda by Nigel Eltringham (chapter 8) and in the post-Soviet countries by Élisabeth Anstett (chapter 9). In doing so, the researchers are led both to explain the scenarios in which the aim is to conceal or disclose the presence of corpses, and to account for their own standpoint at the close or remote distance they choose to maintain. They are also led to consider the psychological, affective or intimate resonances of a strange familiarity with human remains maintained through ethnography.

Thus, this volume aims to launch more than one title. For our study programme, we have built a vast team of researchers working in extremely diverse fields, epochs and scenarios; it seemed vital to make their works accessible through a specific editorial space. We wished to create within Manchester University Press a series of works analysing the fate of the corpses produced from mass violence and genocide. This book series will publish volumes arising from scientific expositions organized in the context of our research programme, standalone collected works and monographs on the subjects linked to the programme. To all of these, the present work aims to serve as an introduction, a programme framework and a methodological manifesto.

Notes

1 B. Bruneteau, *Le Siècle des génocides: violences, massacres et processus génocidaires de l'Arménie au Rwanda* (Paris: Armand Colin, 2004).
2 M. Mazower, *Dark Continent: Europe's Twentieth Century* (Harmondsworth: Penguin, 1999).
3 N. M. Naimark, *Fires of Hatred: Ethnic Cleansing in Twentieth-Century Europe* (Harvard: Harvard University Press, 2001).
4 H. Arendt, *The Origins of Totalitarianism* (New York: Harcourt, Brace, 1951).
5 F. Dikötter, *Mao's Great Famine: The History of China's Most Devastating Catastrophe, 1958–1962* (London: Bloomsbury Publishing, 2010).
6 B. Kiernan, *The Pol Pot Regime: Race, Power, and Genocide in Cambodia Under the Khmer Rouge, 1975–79* (Yale: Yale University Press, 1996).
7 R. Cribb (ed.), *The Indonesian Killings of 1965–1966: Studies from Java and Bali*, Monash Papers on Southeast Asia No. 21 (Clayton: Centre of Southeast Asian Studies, Monash University, 1990).
8 J. P. Chrétien, *Rwanda: les médias du génocide* (Paris: Karthala, 1995).
9 H. Dumas, *Le Génocide au village: le massacre des Tutsi au Rwanda* (Paris: Le Seuil, 2014); S. Totten & E. Markusen, *Genocide in Darfur: Investigating the Atrocities in Sudan* (New York: Routledge, 2006).
10 D. Feierstein, *State Violence and Genocide in Latin America* (New York: Routledge, 2010).

Introduction 7

11 V. Sanford, *Buried Secrets: Truth and Human Rights in Guatemala* (New York: Palgrave Macmillan, 2003).
12 H. Fein, *Genocide: A Sociological Perspective* (London: Sage, 1993); B. Uekert, *Rivers of Blood: A Comparative Study of Government Massacre* (Westport: Praeger Publishers, 1995); A. Alvarez, *Government, Citizens and Genocide: A Comparative and Interdisciplinary Approach* (Bloomington: Indiana University Press, 2001); Y. Ternon, *L'Etat criminel: les génocides au 20e siècle* (Paris: Le Seuil, 1995).
13 For instance, R. J. Van Pelt, *The Case for Auschwitz: Evidence from the Irving Trial* (Bloomington: Indiana University Press, 2002); N. Werth, *L'Ivrogne et la marchande de fleurs: autopsie d'un meurtre de masse 1937–1938* (Paris: Tallandier, 2009).
14 C. Browning, *The Origins of the Final Solution: The Evolution of Nazi Jewish Policy, September 1939–March 1942* (London: Arrow Books, 2005).
15 A. L. Hinton, *Annihilating Difference: The Anthropology of Genocide* (Berkeley: University of California Press, 2002); D. Bloxham, *Genocide on Trial: War Crimes Trials and the Formation of Holocaust History and Memory* (New York: Oxford University Press, 2003).
16 P. Hazan, *Juger la guerre, juger l'histoire: du bon usage des commissions vérité et de la justice internationale* (Paris: Presses Universitaires de France, 2007); E. Barkan, *The Guilt of Nations: Restitution and Negotiating Historical Injustices* (Baltimore: Johns Hopkins University Press, 2000).
17 P. Gray & O. Kendrick (eds), *The Memory of Catastrophe* (Manchester: Manchester University Press, 2004).
18 R. Lemkin, *Axis Rule in Occupied Europe* (Washington: Carnegie Endowment for International Peace, Division of International Law, 1944); W. Schabas, *Genocide in International Law* (Cambridge: Cambridge University Press, 2000).
19 B. Kiernan & R. Gellately, *Specter of Genocide: Mass Murder in Historical Perspective* (Cambridge: Cambridge University Press, 2003); M. Shaw, *War and Genocide: Organized Killing in Modern Society* (Cambridge: Polity Press, 2003); M. Levene, *Genocide in the Age of the Nation State* (London: I. B. Tauris, 2005).
20 B. Schmidt & I. Schröder, *Anthropology of Violence and Conflict* (London: Routledge, 2001); A. L. Hinton & K. L. O'Neill, *Genocide: Truth, Memory and Representation* (Durham: Duke University Press, 2009).
21 A. Corbin, J.-J. Courtine & G. Vigarello, *Histoire du corps* (3 vols) (Paris: Le Seuil, 2005, 2005, 2006); P. Duret & P. Roussel, *Le Corps et ses sociologies* (Paris: Armand Colin, 2005); D. Le Breton, *Anthropologie du corps et modernité* (Paris: Presses Universitaires de France, 1993).
22 T. Shevory, *Body/Politics: Studies in Reproduction, Production and (Re)Construction* (Westport: Praeger, 2000); M. Foucault, 'The birth of social medicine', in J. Faubion (ed.), *Power: Essential Works of Michel Foucault* (New York: New Press, 2000), vol. 3, p. 137.

23 C. Rigeade, *Les Sépultures de catastrophe: approche anthropologique des sites d'inhumations en relation avec des épidémies de peste, des massacres de population et des charniers militaires* (BAR International, 1695; Oxford: Archaeopress, 2007); M. Signoli, D. Chevé, P. Adalian, G. Boëtsch & O. Dutour, *La Peste: entre épidémies et sociétés* (Florence: Firenze University Press, 2007); M. Signoli, 'Archéo-anthropologie funéraire et épidémiologie', *Socio-anthropologie*, 22 (2008), pp. 107–22; K. Verdery, *The Political Lives of Dead Bodies: Reburial and Postsocialist Change* (New York: Columbia University Press, 1999).
24 L.-V. Thomas, *Le Cadavre: de la biologie à l'anthropologie* (Brussels: Éditions Complexe, 1980); G. Clavandier, *Sociologie de la mort: vivre et mourir dans la société contemporaine* (Paris: Armand Colin, 2009).
25 A. Becker, 'Exterminations: le corps et les camps', in G. Vigarello (ed.), *Histoire du corps. Volume 3: Les mutations du regard. Le XXe siècle* (Paris: Editions du Seuil, 2006), pp. 321–39.
26 See the programme's website at www.corpsesofmassviolence.eu (accessed 27 March 2013).
27 N. Eltringham, *Accounting for Horror: Post Genocide Debates in Rwanda* (London: Pluto Press, 2004).
28 A. Y. Guillou, 'An alternative memory of the Khmer Rouge genocide: the ritual treatment of the dead of the mass graves and the killing fields in the Cambodian villages', *South East Asia Research*, 20:2 (2012) (special issue, *Life After Collective Death in South East Asia*), pp. 207–26.
29 S. Garibian, 'Derecho a la verdad. El caso argentino', in R. C. Santiago & V. D. Carlos (eds), *Justicia de transición: el caso de España* (Barcelona: Institut Catala Internacional per la Pau, 2012).
30 Hinton & O'Neill, *Genocide, Truth, Memory and Representation*; Hinton, *Annihilating Difference*.
31 F. Etxeberria, L. H. Erlogorri & Antxon Bandres, *El cementerio de las botellas: enterramientos de presos republicanos en el monte Ezkaba (1942–1945)* (San Sebastian: Sociedad de Ciencias Aranzadi, 2011).
32 J.-M. Dreyfus, 'Conflits de mémoires autour du cimetière de Bergen-Belsen', *Vingtième Siècle: Revue d'Histoire*, 90 (2006), pp. 73–87; A. Korb, *Im Schatten des Weltkriegs: Massengewalt der Ustaša gegen Serben, Juden und Roma in Kroatien 1941–1945* (Hamburg: Hamburg Edition, 2013).
33 C. Fournet, *Genocide and Crimes Against Humanity: Misconceptions and Confusion in French Law and Practice* (Oxford: Hart, 2013).
34 Arendt, *The Origins of Totalitarianism*.
35 P. Hassner, *La Violence et la paix I: de la bombe atomique au nettoyage ethnique* (Paris: Editions Esprit, 1995; Paris: Le Seuil, 2000); P. Hassner, *La Violence et la paix II: la terreur et l'empire* (Paris: Le Seuil, 2003).
36 J. Sémelin, *Purifier ou détruire: usages politiques des massacres et génocides* (Paris: Le Seuil, 2005).

Bibliography

Alvarez, A., *Government, Citizens and Genocide: A Comparative and Interdisciplinary Approach* (Bloomington: Indiana University Press, 2001)

Anstett, É., 'Memory of political repression in post-Soviet Russia: the example of the Gulag', in the *Online Encyclopedia of Mass Violence* (2011), at www.massviolence.org/Memory-of-political-repression-in-post-Soviet-Russia-the

Anstett, É. & L. Jurgenson (eds), *Le Goulag en héritage: pour une anthropologie de la trace* (Paris: Pétra, 2009)

Arendt, H., *The Origins of Totalitarianism* (New York: Harcourt, Brace, 1951)

Barkan, E., *The Guilt of Nations: Restitution and Negotiating Historical Injustices* (Baltimore: Johns Hopkins University Press, 2000)

Becker, A., 'Exterminations: le corps et les camps', in G. Vigarello (ed.), *Histoire du corps. Volume 3: Les mutations du regard. Le XXe siècle* (Paris: Editions du Seuil, 2006), pp. 321–39

Bloxham, D., *Genocide on Trial: War Crimes Trials and the Formation of Holocaust History and Memory* (New York: Oxford University Press, 2003)

Browning, C., *The Origins of the Final Solution: The Evolution of Nazi Jewish Policy, September 1939–March 1942* (London: Arrow Books, 2005)

Bruneteau, B., *Le Siècle des genocides: violences, massacres et processus génocidaires de l'Arménie au Rwanda* (Paris: Armand Colin, 2004)

Chrétien, J. P., *Rwanda: les médias du génocide* (Paris: Karthala, 1995)

Clavandier, G., *Sociologie de la mort: vivre et mourir dans la société contemporaine* (Paris: Armand Colin, 2009)

Corbin, A., J.-J. Courtine & G. Vigarello, *Histoire du corps* (3 vols) (Paris: Le Seuil, 2005, 2005, 2006)

Cribb, R. (ed.), *The Indonesian Killings of 1965–1966: Studies from Java and Bali*, Monash Papers on Southeast Asia No. 21 (Clayton: Centre of Southeast Asian Studies, Monash University, 1990)

Delmas-Marty, M., 'Droit comparé et droit international: interactions et internormativité', in M. Chiavario (ed.), *La Justice pénale internationale entre passé et avenir* (Milan: Giuffre Editore, 2003)

Dikötter, F., *Mao's Great Famine: The History of China's Most Devastating Catastrophe, 1958–1962* (London: Bloomsbury Publishing, 2010)

Dreyfus, J.-M., 'Conflits de mémoires autour du cimetière de Bergen-Belsen', *Vingtième Siècle: Revue d'Histoire*, 90 (2006), pp. 73–87

Dumas, H., *Le Génocide au village: le massacre des Tutsi au Rwanda* (Paris: Le Seuil, 2014)

Duret, P. & P. Roussel, *Le Corps et ses sociologies* (Paris: Armand Colin, 2005)

Eltringham, N., *Accounting for Horror: Post Genocide Debates in Rwanda* (London: Pluto Press, 2004)

Etxeberria, F., L. H. Erlogorri & A. Bandres, *El cementerio de las botellas: enterramientos de presos republicanos en el monte Ezkaba (1942–1945)* (San Sebastian: Sociedad de Ciencias Aranzadi, 2011)

Featherstone, M., M. Hepworth & M. S. Turner (eds), *The Body: Social Process and Cultural Theory* (London: Sage, 1991)

Feierstein, D., *State Violence and Genocide in Latin America* (New York: Routledge, 2010)

Fein, H., *Genocide: A Sociological Perspective* (London: Sage, 1993)

Foucault, M., 'The birth of social medicine', in J. Faubion (ed.), *Power: Essential Works of Michel Foucault* (New York: New Press, 2000), vol. 3, pp. 134–56

Fournet, C., *Genocide and Crimes Against Humanity: Misconceptions and Confusion in French Law and Practice* (Oxford: Hart, 2013)

Garibian, S., 'Derecho a la verdad. El caso argentino', in R. C. Santiago & V. D. Carlos (eds), *Justicia de transición: el caso de España* (Barcelona: Institut Catala Internacional per la Pau, 2012), pp. 51–63

Gray, P. & O. Kendrick (eds), *The Memory of Catastrophe* (Manchester: Manchester University Press, 2004)

Guillou, A. Y., 'An alternative memory of the Khmer Rouge genocide: the ritual treatment of the dead of the mass graves and the killing fields in the Cambodian villages', *South East Asia Research*, 20:2 (2012) (special issue, *Life After Collective Death in South East Asia*), pp. 207–26

Hassner, P., *La Violence et la paix I: de la bombe atomique au nettoyage ethnique* (Paris: Editions Esprit, 1995; Paris: Le Seuil, 2000)

Hassner, P., *La Violence et la paix II: la terreur et l'empire* (Paris: Le Seuil, 2003)

Hazan, P., *Juger la guerre, juger l'histoire: du bon usage des commissions vérité et de la justice internationale* (Paris: Presses Universitaires de France, 2007)

Hinton, A. L., *Annihilating Difference: The Anthropology of Genocide* (Berkeley: University of California Press, 2002)

Hinton, A. L. & K. O'Neill, *Genocide, Truth, Memory and Representation* (Durham: Duke University Press, 2009)

Kiernan, B., *The Pol Pot Regime: Race, Power, and Genocide in Cambodia Under the Khmer Rouge, 1975–79* (Yale: Yale University Press, 1996)

Kiernan, B. & R. Gellately, *Specter of Genocide: Mass Murder in Historical Perspective* (Cambridge: Cambridge University Press, 2003)

Korb, A., *Im Schatten des Weltkriegs: Massengewalt der Ustaša gegen Serben, Juden und Roma in Kroatien 1941–1945* (Hamburg: Hamburg Edition, 2013)

Le Breton, D., *Anthropologie du corps et modernité* (Paris: Presses Universitaires de France, 1993)

Lemkin, R., *Axis Rule in Occupied Europe* (Washington: Carnegie Endowment for International Peace, Division of International Law, 1944)

Levene, M., *Genocide in the Age of the Nation State* (London: I. B. Tauris, 2005)

Mazower, M., *Dark Continent: Europe's Twentieth Century* (Harmondsworth: Penguin, 1999)

Naimark, N. M., *Fires of Hatred: Ethnic Cleansing in Twentieth-Century Europe* (Harvard: Harvard University Press, 2001)

Novick, P., *The Holocaust in American Life* (New York: First Mariner Books, 1999)
Rigeade C., *Les Sépultures de catastrophe: approche anthropologique des sites d'inhumations en relation avec des épidémies de peste, des massacres de population et des charniers militaires* (BAR International, 1695; Oxford: Archaeopress, 2007)
Robben, A., *Death, Mourning, and Burial: A Cross-Cultural Reader* (Oxford: Blackwell, 2004)
Sanford, V., *Buried Secrets: Truth and Human Rights in Guatemala* (New York: Palgrave Macmillan, 2003)
Schabas, W., *Genocide in International Law* (Cambridge: Cambridge University Press, 2000)
Schmidt, B. & I. Schröder, *Anthropology of Violence and Conflict* (London: Routledge, 2001)
Sémelin, J., *Purifier ou détruire: usages politiques des massacres et génocides* (Paris: Le Seuil, 2005)
Shaw, M., *War and Genocide: Organized Killing in Modern Society* (Cambridge: Polity Press, 2003)
Shevory, T., *Body/Politics: Studies in Reproduction, Production and (Re)Construction* (Westport: Praeger, 2000)
Signoli, M., 'Archéo-anthropologie funéraire et épidémiologie', *Socio-anthropologie*, 22 (2008), pp. 107–22, at http://socio-anthropologie.revues.org/1155
Signoli, M., D. Chevé, P. Adalian, G. Boëtsch & O. Dutour, *La peste: entre épidémies et sociétés* (Florence: Firenze University Press, 2007)
Taïeb, E., 'Avant propos: du biopouvoir au thanatopouvoir', *Quaderni*, 62 (2006), pp. 5–15
Ternon, Y., *L'Etat criminel: les génocides au 20e siècle* (Paris: Le Seuil, 1995)
Thomas, L.-V., *Le Cadavre: de la biologie à l'anthropologie* (Brussels: Éditions Complexe, 1980)
Totten, S. & E. Markusen, *Genocide in Darfur: Investigating the Atrocities in Sudan* (New York: Routledge, 2006)
Uekert, B., *Rivers of Blood: A Comparative Study of Government Massacre* (Westport: Praeger, 1995)
Van Pelt, R. J., *The Case for Auschwitz: Evidence from the Irving Trial* (Bloomington: Indiana University Press, 2002)
Verdery, K., *The Political Lives of Dead Bodies: Reburial and Postsocialist Change* (New York: Columbia University Press, 1999)
Werth, N., *L'Ivrogne et la marchande de fleurs: autopsie d'un meurtre de masse 1937–1938* (Paris: Tallandier, 2009)
Wieviorka, A., *Déportation et génocide, entre la mémoire et l'oubli* (Paris: Plon, 1992)

1

The biopolitics of corpses of mass violence and genocide

Yehonatan Alsheh

Introduction

For the past four decades, students of biopolitics have been probing why the spectacular growth in the application of technologies and policies that aim at the optimization of human life has been articulated with a parallel proliferation of human death. Various studies have been suggesting many objects or sites that are arguably highly symptomatic of the issue at hand – a privileged epitome of the biopolitical quandary. The most famous of these is the camp that Giorgio Agamben crowned as the 'biopolitical paradigm of the west',[1] but there are also more mundane objects and sites, such as: archives of biometric data; DNA tests; or the die-hard racial typologies of physical anthropology. This chapter suggests adding corpses of mass violence and genocide to this list.

However, the corpse is not suggested here as yet another privileged object that happens to register all, most or even only some of the mysteries (note the theological slippage) of biopolitics. In fact, as argued below, privileging certain objects or sites within the context of the phenomena concerned, assuming them to somehow be more symptomatic or of primary agency in some underwriting causal scheme, is exactly what a serious look at corpses should help one stop doing.

Corpses of mass violence and genocide, especially when viewed from a biopolitical perspective, force one to focus on the structures of the relations between all that participates in the enfolding case study; to acknowledge and account for the emergent nature of mass violence and genocide; and to loosen and problematize any clear-cut distinction between active and intentional agents and all the inert 'dumb' things through which and on which those actors operate.

Putting together an analytical toolkit for the study of corpses of mass violence and genocide, this chapter looks into what a biopolitical interpretation of mass violence and genocide has brought and may still bring to the table, adding to the already available and productive ideological, behavioural, Marxist, institutional, postcolonial and psychoanalytical interpretations of these phenomena. Noting how little these interpretive frameworks have actually contributed to the study of corpses of mass violence and genocide, this chapter attempts to address the subject matter in view of the remarkable capacity of corpses to resist attempts to reduce them to a mere illustration of a theoretical principle.

The first part of the chapter provides a general introductory outline of the biopolitical approach to the study of genocide and mass violence, pointing out its central problems and limitations. The core problem of the biopolitical approach to genocide research lies in what one may term the correlationist nature of the paradigm. Instead of confronting the actual real phenomena, one is satisfied with musing on the intricacies and aporias of the correlation between a certain consciousness – a certain rationality – a certain thinking collective subject and the constructed reality grasped by this thinking subject. As argued, such a correlationist approach forces a homogenized image of the violence perpetrated, blocking from the very outset any option of opening up to the multiplicity of acts actually perpetrated by various actors who are variously motivated and who target various victim groups.

In view of the criticism detailed in the first part of the chapter, the second part outlines the ways by which the research into corpses of mass violence and genocide is able to support a proper biopolitical analysis of the phenomena concerned. Presenting some of the ideas suggested by the existing research on corpses of mass violence and genocide, this section suggests: (1) a biopolitical interpretation of the agency of corpses in the emergence of the violence, as well as in the aftermath of the violence, from a biopolitical perspective; (2) the historically specific inscription of sovereignty on corpses; (3) the emergent effects of populations of corpses; and (4) the role of forensic anthropology in tapping into corpses as resources for legal and scholarly investigations of mass violence and genocide.

The biopolitical interpretation of genocide and mass violence

Biopolitics, defined in the terms of contemporary social systems theory,[2] is the historically specific structural coupling of the political social system with the biological life system.[3] As of the last decade of the nineteenth century, various scholars, from both the social sciences and the life sciences, have been trying to observe and to effectively theorize the structural coupling of these systems.[4] One may summarize those past 120 years of biopolitical scholarship as suggesting four basic configurations of the concept. These may be tentatively termed: naturalist; politicist; historicist; and ontologist.

The first and earliest configuration – naturalist biopolitics – has two distinct historical versions: a pre-1945 organicist version and an individualistic–behavioural version that emerged in the 1960s. Naturalist biopolitics in both its versions assumes the political to be epiphenomenal and hence in need of being traced back to its underwriting biological determinants and processes. The organist version of naturalist biopolitics assumed collective social entities to be organic wholes that both precede and exceed the individuals composing them.[5] These were termed races or nations and were understood as primordial and organic as oppose to contractual and historically contingent. Politics according to naturalistic biopolitics is essentially derivative – passive manifestations of the internal operations of the biological life system.

The individualist–behaviourist version of naturalist biopolitics and was from its very beginnings in the 1960s fully conscious of the unholy reputation that the organist version had gained since 1945. Hence it deals only with the way that the biology of individual human beings (who are not racially differentiated) underwrites their political behaviour. The individualist–behaviourist version of biopolitics suggests a redeemed version for a biology of politics simply by pinning all that led to (inspired or justified) the abominable policies of the Nazi era on the racist and collectivist premises of the organistic version of naturalist biopolitics. This version of naturalist biopolitics produces studies exploring the way pheromones affect people's choice of candidates in elections; the hard-wiring of human tendencies to prefer their 'own kind' or to dislike the unliked; but also reconstructions of evolutionary mechanisms and circumstances that make people prefer, under certain conditions, authoritarian, repressive regimes to liberal ones.[6]

The second configuration – politicist biopolitics,[7] which emerged in the 1960s and early 1970s – may be presented as advocating the mirror image of naturalist biopolitics, in that it points out the political constitution of the biological life system. Rather than assuming, as naturalist biopolitics does, that the primary operations of the biological life system unilaterally steer the political, this kind of biopolitics observes and theorizes the political regulation and in-depth manipulation of biological life. At the same time it also unveils the thoroughly politicized nature of biological research.

In 1976, Michael Foucault redefined biopolitics, pioneering the third configuration of the concept, which one may term historicist biopolitics.[8] Foucault suggested that the targeting of human life through social and scientific engineering as well as expert administration has been developing since the mid-eighteenth century (a contested periodization which nevertheless parallels Luhmann's periodization of the emergence of modern functionally differentiated social systems).[9]

Rather than trying to discover the biology of politics, or the politics of biology, Foucault argued that one should study the historical development and deployment of multiple strategies and technologies for the political administration of biological life as normalized phenomena. For Foucault, biopolitics came to mean a new form of political power (added to his famous though fuzzy typology of sovereign power, pastoral power and disciplinary power),[10] the object of which is neither the subject (as it is for sovereign power and pastoral power) nor the singular human body (as it is for disciplinary power), but the biological features of human beings as they are measured and aggregated on the level of populations.[11]

Interchangeably using the term 'biopower', Foucault tried to capture the emergent development of technologies of power that address the management of and control over populations. The technologies collected under the title of biopower have been superimposed on top of and around the already pervasive disciplinary technologies of power.

Biopolitics as an emerging new configuration of power was designed to control life and the biological process of humans as species, aiming at regularizing life. Just as with regard to his concept of disciplinary power, by 'biopolitics' Foucault meant a growing and ever more sophisticated apparatus of forecasts, statistical estimates and various means of measurement – an assortment of security mechanisms.

According to Foucault, biopower and disciplinary power operate as two layers or planes of an integrative form of power (biodisciplinary power) that is – arguably – fundamentally different from sovereign power.[12] While sovereign power is deductive in essence (the sovereign takes away either taxes or life), biodisciplinary power fosters, develops and cultivates: it is generative in essence.

Hence, while sovereign power has always been oppressive and mechanistic in nature, biodisciplinary power brought about a completely new way of exercising power: the gradual and elaborate development of the fine art of cultivating self-regulating systems. This emerged out of the vary praxis of disciplinary power, since the creation of various practices and technologies of discipline led to the unavoidable discovery of the limits of coercion. But it also discovered a new frontier: the tuning and optimization of all that is capable of self-regulation (individual humans but also their social systems). Whether referring to various so-called 'technologies of the self', to the market or to populations, the mechanical conception of power (Newtonian mechanics) gives way to statistical phenomena, with their normal and abnormal patterns of distribution.[13] But more importantly, it opened up precious room for fine manipulation, by means of a careful targeting of the margins of normalized phenomena (for example the development of the marginal school in economics).[14]

Elaborating on the difference between sovereign power and biodisciplinary power, Foucault hypothesized that the genocidal potential of biodisciplinary power arises from the historical integration of biodisciplinary power with sovereign power (his famous announcement that we are yet to cut off the king's head).[15] Arguably, genocide comes about once sovereign power's death function (the sovereign's inalienable right to kill) is incorporated into biodisciplinary power as another means for optimizing life – weeding and trimming as functional elements of cultivation.

Tragically, this new biopolitical meaning of death liberates sovereign power's insatiable hunger for death (which modern political philosophy never took seriously enough) from all that used to restrain it beforehand.[16] This suppressed dark essence of sovereignty, which modern biopolitics freed to loom large, informs the fourth configuration of biopolitics, which one may term ontologist biopolitics. This configuration appeared in the last decade of the twentieth century, and consists of the works of various thinkers (some saw it as an Italian school),[17] most famously Giorgio Agamben,[18] Antonio Negri (co-authoring with Michel Hardt)[19] and Roberto Esposito.[20]

This configuration of the concept of biopolitics focuses on the fact that historical experience most clearly and brutally shows that biodisciplinary power has never fostered, nurtured or cultivated all human life. To the contrary, biodisciplinary power was always deployed in a way that optimizes the life of some populations while abandoning, when not actively sacrificing, the life of other populations. Biodisciplinary power has always operated as if there is an unwritten rule that the optimization of the life of certain populations justifies (when not necessitating) the exposure of other populations to less than optimal conditions, and even the killing of them. The question is of course why? And what is one to make of it?

One may begin by noting that biodisciplinary power has never been deployed in the service of humanity's universal interest, due to the unfortunate inexistence of a collective actor embodying such an interest. Hardt and Negri seems to be the only theoreticians of ontological biopolitics believing in the very possibility of such an actor, while the others follow Carl Schmitt in insisting on the ontological impossibility of an all-inclusive political community (the act of exclusion as the constitutive act of political communities).[21]

While biodisciplinary power was never all-inclusive in its operations, either contingently so or out of principle, it was developed by and in the service of states – the modern colonial nation-state.[22] These states have always been governed by certain population groups (the ruling classes, national groups whose nation-state it was) as a means for dominating other populations (the exploited masses, colonized peoples).

But what has informed this discriminatory and unequal deployment of biodisciplinary power since the mid-eighteenth century (or any alternative periodization that may be suggested)? How is it decided which lives are worth living – worthy of optimization – and which are not, or even which are in need of extermination, so that the worthy life will be optimized? If life itself is the ultimate and only source of value (as developed by thinkers of *Lebensphisolophie* since the second half of the nineteenth century),[23] then where did the notion of life that is not good – life not worth living – come from?

While naturalist biopolitics will trace the origin of this distinction to the biological life system (inter-racial hatred, evolutionary aversion towards unfit lives and so forth), and politicist biopolitics will trace it to the political social system (the interest of some collective actor), historicist biopolitics will suggest the historical emergence of this distinction as part of the restructuring of the coupling of the systems. More specifically, as already mentioned, it was the integration of sovereign power with biodisciplinary power. Foucault combined this process with a proposed genealogy of racism (unfortunately, or even symptomatically as some less charitable minds may argue, an all too Euro-centric one and hence somewhat garbled). The core issue, however, is that the integration of sovereign power and biodisciplinary power was premised (most clearly from the second half of the nineteenth century) on an essentially conflictual social ontology – a social ontology in which social groups, either races or classes, struggle throughout history.

Sovereignty in this regard must be understood as essentially partisan – given to one social group to be used against another. Simply put, historicist biopolitics suggests that while sovereign power's death function used to be a communicative gesture – a way to state who is sovereign – the emergence of biodisciplinary power enabled the sovereign social group to optimize its own life by means of minimalizing the life of its adversary (or assumed to be adversary) social group.

Ontological biopolitics attempts to elaborate this historical emergence of the distinction between life worthy of living and life unworthy of living by accentuating its negative normative value. Whether embodied in the trans-historical figure of the homo sacer, empire's radically novel mode of subjugation in postmodern times, or the result of a constitutive immunizing logic that political philosophy has not yet transcended, the structural coupling of biological life and the political social system is ontologically flawed. It is so in the sense that it is not just a contingent abusive modality of this structural coupling – a bad version within a variety of already available alternatives: in these pre-messianic times, nothing escapes this flaw.[24]

Ontological biopolitics differs from the other configurations of the concept by being thoroughly normative in approach. Ontological biopolitics constructs its concept around what is understood to be the biopolitical production of evil, even radical evil in the case of Agamben and Esposito – genocide. As Thomas Lemke and others argued, for Agamben biopolitics is above all 'thenatopolitics'.[25]

Problems with the biopolitical interpretation

One can point out three basic problems with the biopolitical interpretation of genocide and mass violence. The first is the tendency to present a genocidal interpretation of biopolitics rather than biopolitical interpretations of genocide.

It so happens that up until now the literature on biopolitics and genocide has been mostly written by theoreticians who were far more interested in (and informed about) biopolitics than in genocide as their main object of enquiry. Rather than using biopolitics as an analytical perspective or a toolkit for the study of mass violence and genocide, providing new insights and developing new research agendas, it was the historical occurrence of genocide, or a very particular representation of it, to be exact, that was invoked as laying bare the nature and meaning of modern biopolitics.

Genocide in fact becomes in ontological biopolitical literature a manifestation, a negative revelation, most notably in the literature musing on the inconceivability of the Holocaust,[26] of biopolitics' alleged inner essence, which one should uncover and acknowledge. The various intersections between the biopolitics of genocide and the political theology of genocide should not be overlooked, yet at the same time one should avoid an uncritical slippage from one to the other. The more grotesque versions of this argument, in which one is called to somehow acknowledge that there is no noteworthy difference between a United Nations refugee camp and a Nazi extermination camp, have been sufficiently criticized.[27]

However, even in its more subtle and nuanced versions (for example as presented by Roberto Esposito and Achille Mbembe), the actual historical phenomenon to which the concept of genocide is meant to refer is forced into a process of growing abstraction, so that it may indeed be revealed at the heart of every act of modern biopolitical sovereignty and not only when a genos is actually being destroyed. Soon, what is left of genocide is its moral severity, its being a non-contested manifestation of radical evil, an exclamation mark in the middle of an otherwise endless flux of indifferent and undifferentiated eventuation – the one consensual example of the bad polis, in view of a complete inability to stabilize any argument regarding the nature of the good polis.

As Dirk A. Moses powerfully argued with regard to the literature analysing the relation between genocide and modernity, upon which biopolitical interpretations of genocide heavily rely, the analysis of genocide as symptomatic of modernity has unjustifiably focused on the Holocaust, while disregarding genocidal campaigns that took place in the colonial context.[28]

In order to assume the exceptionality of the Nazi genocidal projects, one needs to forget not only colonial precedents but also the destruction of Armenian and other Christian populations in Ottoman Anatolia during the First World War. Much of the high-pitched disillusionment expressed by many intellectuals in the aftermath of the Second World War, which ontological biopolitics still carries on, is the unflattering result of Euro-centric navel gazing. All too ironically, students of ontological biopolitics wish to present the Nazi horror as symptomatic of biopolitics in all its expressions, yet the drama of the provocation is based on unveiling a deeply hidden symmetry between the two great opposing camps of the Second World War. This in turn is meant to prove the power of the in-depth philosophical analysis practised by students of ontological biopolitics. However, much of this seems to collapse once the unsettling effect of the discovery is revealed to be nothing but the sad outcome of the parochialism that is of course the true meaning of Euro-centrism.

This leads us to the second problem with the biopolitical paradigm in genocide research, which was already pointed out in Dan Stone's account of this approach.[29] Appreciative of the insights provided by the biopolitical approach to genocide research, and its obvious effectiveness in inspiring scholarly attention to and writing on the subject of genocide, from disciplines other than history, Stone also showed that this approach, though unfortunately ignorant of the centrality of colonial genocide in the historical emergence of this phenomenon, is nevertheless compatible with the findings of current research concerning colonial genocide. Stone notes a certain resemblance between the so-called functionalist school in Holocaust historiography and the biopolitical approach.[30] He argues that the biopolitical approach and the functionalist school share the same unjustified disregard of the role played by: irrational ideology; primordial fantasies of violence; dynamics of contamination and sacrificial cleansing; and regeneration and redemption via violence and transgression. These atavistic irrationalities, as opposed to the common and symptomatic mentality of political modernity advocated by the biopolitical approach, were completely historically contingent, budding and flourishing in certain political cultures while being weeded out in others.

The biopolitical approach, it may be argued, explains why genocide can take place, yet it does not answer why it usually does not. This also sheds some light on ontological biopolitics' insistence on a hidden (or not, as it sometimes surfaces) genocidal core in all modern biopolitical regimes. However, one may also choose, instead of arguing that genocide is somehow universally characteristic of all biopolitical regimes, to point out the historically singular elements responsible for the activation of genocidal potentials in modern biopolitical regimes.

One would not have been so perplexed by this stubborn insistence on a genocidal interpretation of biopolitics if there was not so much to be gained from a biopolitical interpretation of genocide. An illuminating example of a fruitful perspective that historicist biopolitics may open up, leading to a better understanding of the historical phenomenon of genocide, can be found in Foucault's claim that:

> this power to kill, which ran through the entire social body of Nazi society, was first manifested when the power to take life and death, was granted not only to the state but to a whole series of individuals, to a considerable number of people (such as the SA and the SS and so on). Ultimately, everyone in the Nazi State had the power of life and death over his or her neighbors, if only because of the practice of informing, which effectively meant doing away with the people next door, or having them done away with.[31]

The above argument, once one moves beyond reading it as nothing but a contribution to the analytics of modern political power, leads one to look into what the historian Christian Gerlach called the participatory nature of the violence in cases of mass violence and genocide.[32] While the term 'mass violence' is commonly understood as referring to the massive number of victims, Gerlach pointed out that in most of the relevant historical case studies the number of perpetrators involved is also massive.

However, one should beware of bracketing away the participatory nature of the violence by simply homogenizing the perpetrating multitude with the assumption that they all had the same intentions, the same understanding of all that was going on, the same motivation for doing what they were doing, the same image of the victimized populations, the same criterion for selection of victims and the concrete violent acts actually performed, and so forth. Instead, one should acknowledge the substantial variation within the perpetrating multitudes, which empirical findings have so exhaustively indicated. Acknowledging this variation leads, as Gerlach so powerfully showed, to a strikingly different image of mass violence and genocide.

Although, as Gerlach's work itself shows, written documents do not exclusively represent the perspective of the political centre but also its various negotiations with the scattered on-the-ground actors, there is nevertheless a certain homogenizing bias to written documentation that the researcher must read against, maintaining the hermeneutics of suspicion.

The growing use of oral history in the study of mass violence and genocide, and its constant methodological sophistication, has, to a point, countered this problem of written documentation. However, there is much to be said for the role corpses as a source for reconstructing the heterogeneous reality that takes place at the ground level of perpetration.

While written documents provide one with the way things should have happened, as framed by the perspective of those producing the documentation, corpses document – albeit partially and in a fragmented way – what was actually done to the victimized populations. In this regard one may even suggest that corpses constitute an almost privileged site of evidence with regard to the realities of participatory violence, as opposed to traditional archival sources that bracket away the core significance of the fact that certain kinds of violence are participatory in nature.

The third (and one may suggest the most severe) problem is that biopolitics, at the height of its theoretical sophistication, that is, biopolitics of the Foucauldian historicist kind, is thoroughly correlationist in its approach. The term 'correlationism' was suggested by Quentin Meillassoux in 2006,[33] as referring to any current of thought maintaining that one only ever has access to the correlation between thinking and reality and never to either of these considered apart from the other. Meillassoux argues that twentieth-century correlationism focused on language and/or consciousness as the medium of the correlation between the alleged 'thinking subject' and the 'thought-of object'.

Turning back to the subject at hand, historicist biopolitics indeed identifies and analyses the historical emergence of a distinct kind of political consciousness (mentality) embodied in/produced by language – a distinct political rationality embodied in/produced by discourse and an elaborate apparatus of discipline and security technologies and practices.

Foucault is in fact the most influential example in continental philosophy of the second half of the twentieth century for strong correlationism, in which the thoroughly contingent nature of the correlation is pushed to its most radical conclusion.[34] Foucault's biopolitics (as well as his analyses of disciplinary power and technologies of the self) should be understood as continuing the corporalization of Kant's transcendental subject, following the work of Martin Heidegger and its influential development in the thought of Morris Merleau-Ponty. The thinking subject is completely embodied, that is to say thoroughly constrained and conditioned by the biological and social systems of which the subject is merely an emergent effect.

However, while Foucault was only drawing conclusions from the corporality of the thinking subject, by suggesting that the historical emergence of disciplinary and later on biopolitical societies necessarily led to the production of subjectivities whose correlation with whatever is thought of has been dramatically restructured, he also brought about (though never noting it himself) the collapse of correlationism.[35]

By labouring to reconstruct an entire typology of different structures of correlation between thinking subjects and thought-of objects (though the result may be criticized in retrospect for being grossly generalized, Euro-centric and arbitrary) Foucault confessed the absolute nature of contingency, not only of the correlation but in fact also of reality itself – the contingent nature of reality itself, regardless of the presence of absence of anyone thinking it.

Exactly because different subjectivities are emergent effects of different biological and social systems (which in turn continue to vary in their historically specific structural coupling), one must admit that there have been and still will one day be biological and maybe even social systems that did not and will not produce any subjectivities at all.

Often throughout the last seventy years, people have imagined the coming of a society that will bring humanity to its end. Such a nuclear, ecological or what-have-you apocalypse will be as real as it gets, even if, afterwards, there is no longer anyone to witness it, that is, to be its correlate by thinking it.[36] Just as an apocalyptic future reality will exist even though there is no subjectivity to think it, so the reality that existed before the first biological and social systems to produce a thinking subjectivity emerged with whatever structure of correlation to a thought-of world.

The correlationism of biopolitics has led to the interpretation of genocide as a possible manifestation (a most symptomatic one) of a correlation between a historically specific political subjectivity – to be sure, a collective subjectivity – and a political reality that neither precedes nor derives from the political subjectivity experiencing it. One cannot consider the historical reality of genocide without the biopolitical rationality thinking it, which is the very point ontological biopolitics constantly makes.

At the same time, one cannot contemplate biopolitics without genocide. And that is exactly where the problem is. This correlationist approach denies from the very outset one's ability to be surprised by historical reality, which is, after all, always more complex and other than it is thought to be. Just as the excesses of reality are declared from the very outset to be unintelligible, so are the excesses of the other side of the correlation. It also denies a meaningful plurality of thinking subjects – a viable assemblage of only partially compatible perspectives, each operating within a different political rationality.

Hence this correlationist approach ends up forcing a false homogeneity on the actual historical occurrence of genocide. This homogeneity is forced on all components of the phenomenon: the perpetrators, who are assumed to be a homogenized mass of actors operating within the same single political rationality; the victims, who are assumed to be a homogenized mass of 'bare lives'; and the genocidal acts themselves, which are assumed to be killing or the intentional bringing about of exposure to death.

Gerlach showed how such a homogenized conception of genocide prevents research accounting for what is in fact a non-focal multiplicity in which a variety of different perpetrator groups target in many different ways and for many different reasons a variety of victim groups. The situation is extremely variable overtime and across territories.

However, biopolitics is in no way necessarily correlationist. In order to continue the study of the biopolitics of various phenomena in a non-correlationist way, all that one needs to do is to turn from the study of the historically specific structure of the correlation to the study of the historically specific structure of the coupling between the political social system and the biological life system.

Populations of corpses

A good way to begin substantializing this suggested turn from the study of structures of correlation to the study of the structures of the coupling of the systems is to re-examine Dan Stone's aforementioned criticism of biopolitics' blindness to genocide's irrational, carnivalesque, sacrificial and liminal dimensions. Stone stressed the ideological origins of these aspects, aiming at a description of the perpetrators' collective consciousness, which is of course a thoroughly correlationist approach to this issue. However, one can just as much address the production of this unworldly atmosphere, that profound and uncanny sense of a time and place that are out of time and displaced, with its far-reaching effects on prevailing taboos and people's sense of what they can and cannot – may and may not – should and should not – do, 'from below'. That is to say, one can try to understand how that horrible carnivalesque and liminal ambiance emerges from the bare and physical presence of corpses 'on the ground': sensually there, in all their revolting and nauseating potency (noting Sartre's invocation of nausea as the somatic sensation of estranging oneself from the subterranean taken-for-granted instrumental 'tool-being' of things).[37]

The ways by which the bare presence of corpses seems to contribute dramatically to an escalation in the violence perpetrated has in fact been pointed out in many empirical case studies (one such is presented in chapter 5). The interaction between the physical presence of the corpses (in its most direct sensual sense, the sight of death, the smell of death) and certain – alleged – primordial deep layers of consciousness in humans, a speculated deep-seated aversion to and terror in the presence of embodied death, has also received noteworthy attention, as Finn Stepputat critically outlines.[38]

Understanding the corpse as the ultimate signifier of death, certain psychoanalysts pointed to the emergence of the primordial and omnipresent fear of death (assumed to be the originary form and ultimate meaning of all other fears) as an explanation for corpses' emotive capacities. However, as long as one indeed argues that the corpse is understood by all people at all times and in all cultures as the ultimate fearsome signifier of death, the presence of which causes all people to react in certain ways, one is subject to all the aforementioned limitations of naturalistic biopolitics.

In fact, by arguing that a corpse is a signifier (let alone an ultimate one), whether of death or of anything else, one is missing much of the point here. Joost Fontein pointedly suggests explaining at least some of the potency of corpses by noting that corpses appear impossibly to be both person and object – or just as impossibly neither person nor object. In any case, the corpse is a site where this constitutive distinction most effectively malfunctions.[39]

In other words, rather than being signifiers of anything, corpses bring about (but do not represent!) a collapse of signification, which in such cases (as opposed to art or other contexts of well contained ecstasy) is not pleasant but rather ghastly and uncanny. Julia Kristeva in this regard, building on the work of George Bataille and Merry Douglas, suggested understanding the corpse as the ultimate 'abject', by which she meant a pre-objectified 'thing' whose radical exclusion constitutes one's subjectivity, and whose forced presence threatens to collapse one back into a pre-subjective mess.[40]

This speculative explanation has its limitations of course – it is not entirely clear how Kristeva evades falling into the naturalistic assumption that all this somehow applies to all people at all times and in all cultures. However, it can be interpreted as dealing with the dynamic of real interactions that precede the emergence of a thinking subject and thought-of objects (before the successful exclusion of the abject) and what may still happen after the collapse (the failure of the exclusion) of the correlation between the subject and the object.

Moreover, Kristeva's theory of abjection suggests looking into the complex way by which correlational aspects and non-correlational aspects interact and coexist. For example, it suggests looking into exactly when the presence of bare corpses disrupts the stable structure of an existing correlation between a given subjectivity and its world, bringing forth the detailed ways in which the real structural coupling of the political social system and the biological life system (but also other couplings of systems of course) still condition, constrain and pattern the havoc of the over-flooding abjection.

One often reads about the unsettling effects of the abject, and more specifically about the way that the corpse unsettles the distinction between a person and thing. However, it seems that very little is actually explained or even described by the adjective 'unsettled'. Interestingly, Fontein widely refers to unsettled spirits that haunt Zimbabweans, demanding the exhumation of their bones from foreign lands and their proper burial in their ancestral land.[41] However, while it is clear what will settle those angry spirits and how this may be accomplished (repatriation of the bones and their proper burial), it is completely unclear what may settle the unsettled distinction between person and object in the case of the corpse. In fact, by using the term 'unsettled' to describe the corpses' effect on the distinction between person and object, one unjustifiably smuggles in an expectation for a resettlement of the distinction.

The abject in general, and corpses more concretely, indeed seem to uproot one from a secure and immersed being in and with the world. Yet what do corpses do when they are said to unsettle? In the terms suggested by Graham Harman, they may be said to confront one with the ontological drama of the reversal between the interacting accessible systems and their withdrawn abyssal depths, insular and singular as they ever-elusively are.[42]

By declaring certain effects to be unsettling, one is missing out on the chance to point out the reality (fleeting and elusive though it is) of things. It is this exact dynamic of limited disruption – bounded and always partially structured malfunction of sense – that corpses may (only may) force on some of those co-present with them. It is this dynamic that brings forth the excess that everything always hold in reserve. This excess is inaccessible and as such an unknowable-unknown, yet its existence is grounded in the absolute contigency of it all.

The above collapses of meaning lead to Stone's horrid sanguinary carnival, taking place within reality and as such produced by it (for example through the physical presence of corpses). But just as importantly they are conditioned, constrained and patterned by it. Although there is no reason to assume that all the actors know and understand all that indeed goes on (as simplistic ideology-centred explanations uncritically assume), or that all actors involved are somehow sufficiently similar to be regarded as thinking the same (a criticism applying to all existing theoretical understandings of genocide, save that suggested by Gerlach), the variation among the actors involved is nevertheless still constrained by the reality of the situation.

Hence, a typology of being with corpses traceable in the various case studies of genocide and mass violence is called for. Such a typology would be able to differentiate, for example, between –

- bounded sites of mass slaughter over a relatively short duration, such as:
    - the prototypical modern battlefield with its dense distribution of living survivors, dead corpses but also substantial numbers of people in 'inbetween' states, such as people with wounds of various degrees of severity, and some portions of scattered bodily matter (dismembered organs, blood etc.)
    - the slaughter pits and massacre sites in which the murdered victims are piled within a mass grave, often sheltering a few survivors who manage to hide (or being unconscious are presumed dead) among the corpses, all in the presence of the perpetrators and those physically producing the site (digging the grave, piling the corpses and so forth)
- bounded sites in which mass death occurs over more extended durations such as:
    - the detainment/concentration/labour camp, with its high mortality rate due to starvation, exposure, epidemics, where

corpses function as a biohazard, greatly exasperating the spread of epidemics
  - the industrialized killing factory, in which the high-pressure slaughter characteristic of the battlefield and the slaughter pit takes place almost daily over a long duration of time
- normal, 'everyday life' sites turned sites of mass death such as:
  - the village
  - the urban setting
  - the bombarded area
- but also non-bounded sites of mass death over extended time spans, in which the survivors are forced to move on, leaving the corpses behind, such as the trail marched during forced expulsions and death marches
- and last but far from being least, societies on their own territory in the aftermath of a conflict, facing the state-sponsored, accidental or purposeful resurfacing of corpses and mass graves.

The above is of course also historically specific – parading its absolute contingency in the restructurings that the passing of time forces.[43] It also meaningfully intersects with political theology (the historically specific structural coupling of the political social system with the religious social system). Corpses of mass violence and genocide are highly capable of producing religious experiences, whether of the presence of the horrific sublime or of the shattering loss of all faith in a benevolent Almighty, and any other possible formulation.

Bataille's speculative analysis of the relations between death, its embodiment in the corpse and the political phenomenon of sovereignty well exceeds the use Kristeva made of certain elements in his theory. However, Bataille appears to suggest tracing the political back to its alleged religious underpinnings, not only explaining away the coupling of the systems by understanding the political social system as epiphenomenal to the religious social system, but in fact denying the very differentiation of those systems from each other. In this regard Charles Taylor rightly points out that Bataille is completely premodern.[44]

This is of course also the problem, since corpses cannot be understood without noting the profound historicity of the very distinction between life and death that corpses so effectively embody. The ultimate radicalization of the distinction, in which life became everything while death became nothing but a limit concept – the utter nothing that life negates – is relatively recent, emerging only in the second half of the nineteenth century with the aforementioned *Lebensphilosophie*.

As the distinction between life and death has often been suggested to run parallel to the distinction between heaven and earth – the godly realm and the human realm – immanence and transcendence, it is hardly surprising that the radicalization of the distinction between life and death went hand in hand with the radicalization of the distinction between immanence (becoming nothing less than all that is) and transcendence (so fundamentally non-existent that the mere notion is declared unintelligible) at about the same time. However, one cannot avoid wondering whether the fact that the corpse is so inconveniently something, as opposed to an embodiment of radical nothingness, does not suggest yet another dimension to the abjection its bare presence causes.

Certain corpses and even mere fragments of certain corpses came to be regarded in a dramatically different way during the late fourth and fifth centuries, with the rise of the cult of saints in Latin Christianity.[45] Peter Brown in his classic study of this phenomenon suggested interpreting this rising tendency to worship not only the graves of certain holy figures but also their bare bodily remains (often in the form of actually touching and kissing them) as signifying a radical change in the function of the dead and the cemetery in the crumbling Roman world.[46] Beyond moving the dead and their site of burial to the very centre of the city, and their constitution as one of the Church's cardinal forms of capital, the corpse was assumed to retain in a very significant way its link with the soul. Adopting and deeply reinterpreting the Jewish conception of the resurrection of the dead, the corpse was now understood as an unfolding drama (at a somewhat glacial pace, obviously): a reversal between its decaying dead surface and its withdrawn, heavenly depths, from which the soul and with it resurrected life will re-emerge once kingdom come.

In fact, it was exactly because the corpse's life withdraws into the invisible and inaccessible substratum that the corpse was identified as a privileged gateway to that inaccessible transcendence. Rather than unbearably embodying the distinction between life and death, the cult of the saints presents a substantial period in which western Christianity assumed the corpse to be the blessed and most joyous place where this distinction appears ephemeral.

This historicity of the corpse and the distinction between life and death is deeply related to the rise of modern biopolitics. In presenting his account of the historical emergence of the modern structural coupling of the political social system and the biological life system, Foucault underlined a profound change in the meaning of death around the early eighteenth century. Death used to be a great public moment of transition, as the dying abandoned their particular direct sovereign in this world and were surrendered to the ultimate sovereign of all. Death used to be a spectacular moment of affirmation – the dying individual was finally brought to justice – the fearsome divine ruling that each individual was advised to carefully expect finally came. Life used to be, in this sense, nothing but a fleeting duration in which the individual might have succeeded in temporarily escaping sovereign power, to sin without immediate punishment. Death affirmed that there is no escape, and that the real sovereign – the Almighty – patiently yet surely waits.

This meaning of death gained prominence in western Christendom only from the thirteenth century onwards, gradually replacing the one briefly sketched above. This new meaning of death is traceable in various paintings, inscriptions and sculptures of corpses being eaten by worms, the skeleton hidden beneath the flesh and other grim representations of death as the ultimate truth of life.[47] It is only from then onwards that one may speak of the horrifying quality of corpses, now emanating from their function as signifiers (not embodiments!) of the fearsome divine judgement that waits all after their death. Interestingly, as for example Fontein shows with regard to current-day Zimbabwe, certain societies prefer to keep corpses lying in shallow mass graves, or any other form of inappropriate burial, so that they may be used as evidence once (or should) the political constellation enable the establishment of a court (either international or national).[48] It seems that though today corpses no longer represent the inescapable final and just judgement of the Almighty (at least not necessarily), an awaited just trial is still somehow inscribed on them – figuring on a horizon they open.

As mentioned, Foucault characterized premodern sovereign power as a deductive mode of power, a subtracting power that takes away (whether taxes or freedom or life). The losses created by the exercise of power are awesome monuments to its potent presence, just as execution and the collection of taxes are ceremonial gestures of its sovereignty. Modern biopower, on the other hand, is a generative, cultivating power that seeks to stimulate, enhance, accelerate, better, regulate and normalize its object of concern – human populations. Rather than taking life or allowing to live, biopower fosters life or disallows it to the point of death – it is a power that makes populations live and hence can just let certain populations die.

This of course entails a substantial change in the meaning of death. Rather than monuments to the potency of the sovereign, death becomes either failure – proof of impotency – or a testimony of absence: where biopower is not doing its job, because of intentional abandonment but also non-intentional state collapse.

With the advent of modern biopolitics, death, rather than ending all impunity as the dead person was surrendered to the Almighty, became the moment at which the individual finally and irreversibly escaped power (as in the frustrating suicide of the offender before the court had the chance to sentence her or him to death).[49] As such, death became the absolute moment of annihilation, power's absolute limit.

Death, argued Foucault, changed from a most public spectacle of affirmed and inescapable pan sovereignty to the most private moment imaginable: that which no one could witness, not even the dying man himself.[50] The living body came to be understood in the age of the subject as the literal embodiment of subjectivity, that which communicates the otherwise secluded psychic system – it is through the body that the consciousness accesses the world, as well as being accessed itself.

The living body negates in this regard the privacy of consciousness, which is why its death results in a terminal moment of absolute privacy. An absolute privacy, which seems to be unbearably violated when the corpse is laid bare – pornographically (as western discourse tends to term it) exposed.

Yet, the above picture of a persecuting power, roaring in frustration around the corpse which by dying managed to escape, is of course also misleading. After all, why would modern biopolitics be frustrated when some lives cross over its ultimate limit, that is, die? All too often, chasing those lives away is deemed necessary for the prosperity if not outright survival of other lives.

As mentioned, historicist biopolitics and afterwards ontological biopolitics diagnosed the working of a reason advocating that the survival of certain populations necessitates the extinction of certain other populations. This often appears in a weaker version: the prosperity and well-being of certain populations justifies the exposure or abandonment of some other populations. Death is as bureaucratically planned and organized as life. Because of the political power to generate and preserve gross inequality in the distribution of access to resources, services and risk-free and pathogen-free environments, it is possible to cultivate some healthy and prosperous populations.

Yet the above also stipulates the managed disposal of corpses, not just for reasons of hygiene but also because the production of death as one of the means by which the good life or certain populations is produced is better kept away from sight, or at least under the pretence of complete control. The corpse as the embodiment of death appears in modernity as always also subversive, while populations of corpses have the effect of spreading so much subversion that they create the nightmarish horrid carnivalesque atmosphere mentioned above, with its profound unruliness.

It is in this context that one needs also to consider and to understand the work of forensic anthropologists on exhumed human remains in the aftermath of mass violence and genocide since the mid-1980s onwards.[51] The truly Promethean attempt to identify each corpse and trace it back as much as possible to a concrete perpetrator and on-the-ground event, while obviously motivated by the desire for justice and closure[52] for the surviving relatives, is also meant to reconstitute the spectacle of political control over death and to defuse all subversive effects that those corpses may still unleash.[53]

A cardinal characteristic of corpses of mass violence and genocide is the trivial fact that there are so many of them, both widespread and in large concentrations. The specifically modern structural coupling of the political system and the biological life system can be modelled via the notion of populations as self-regulating collective entities with emergent properties. Emerging properties appear (activated, actualized) only when the various units composing those populations interact with one another.[54] Put simply, large concentrations of corpses are far more – and significantly different – than the mere sum of individual corpses. One is hence called to study the characteristics and implications of corpses as populations – the various emerging effects of large concentrations of corpses in their various patterns of distribution across time and space.

To start with, populations of corpses constitute a biohazard, generating epidemics that dramatically increase mortality, as seen in various case studies.[55] Hence several detailed typologies are called for in which the various case studies are sorted into those in which epidemics played a central role in increasing mortality rates, and those in which this was less so (or not at all) the case. The evidence suggests the latter is in fact a practically empty category – despite the image of an efficient, 'clean', industrialized extermination advocated by certain biopolitical interpretations of genocide.

Given that, one is required to outline the various ways by which people, from the victimized groups, third parties or perpetrators, neutralize – or fail to neutralize – this biohazard: by means of traditional methods; by means of modern technology and logistics; or under the stringent conditions of acute emergency.

Another typology stemming from a focus on the emerging effects of populations of corpses consists of classifying all the ways in which people (again, perpetrators, other victims or third parties) extract resources out of large concentrations of corpses: from jewellery and other on-the-body valuables (gold teeth, but in this day and age also the harvesting of organs) to hair, fat (the infamous soap production rumour) and finally (ultimately?) cannibalism.[56]

As mentioned, since the mid-1980s and increasingly with every decade that passes, corpses become a resource for both legal and scholarly investigations. Populations of corpses are in this regard planes of inscription, documenting some of what was actually perpetrated. Far from displaying the clean, dispassionate, efficient and uniform killing advocated by some biopolitical conceptions of genocide, one finds an entire repertoire of variations and excesses.

On the corpses one finds the traces of the various kinds of perpetrating groups who targeted those people for various reasons, in various circumstances and by various kinds of violence.[57] In this regard, corpses put forward the noteworthy plurality of what actually happens, as opposed to the homogenic state-sponsored project envisioned by ideological schemes and pretences.

How, given the above, is one to understand the biopolitics of forensic anthropology, which is the main discipline specializing in the contextual interpretation of corpses? Is it premised (as seems to be the case) on an intuitive suspicion of naturalistic biopolitical assumptions? If so, is it necessarily so, and if not, what kind of biopolitics underpins forensic anthropology?

An enquiry in the biopolitics of forensic anthropology is also called for because it is currently one of the key disciplines that confront the problem of race – a cardinal example of a biopolitical problem, which of course has a deep association with genocide and many manifestations of mass violence.

On the one hand, the American Association of Physical Anthropologists stated in its 1996 *Statement on Biological Aspects of Race* that: 'Humanity cannot be classified into discrete geographical categories with absolute boundaries';[58] and the American

Anthropological Association argued in its 1998 *Statement on Race* that: 'it has become clear that human populations are not unambiguously clearly demarcated, biologically distinct groups'.[59]

On the other hand, in a conference organized by the American Association of Physical Anthropologists held in New Mexico in May 2007, on the issue of race, the so-called 'geneticist' camp (advocating that human genetic variation does not support racial classification) was challenged by a so-called 'morphologist' camp, which argued that: 'worldwide geographic patterning in cranial form does produce observable regional patterns and that, although these flow into one another, there are some fairly distinct clusters'.[60]

The lingering – diehard – insistence on the actual biological existence of something similar enough to that category called race is fuelled in the field of physical anthropology by the practice of forensic anthropologists whose position is well explained by Conrad B. Quintyn, an associate member of the American Academy of Forensic Sciences: 'When I began to assist law enforcement in identifying human skeletal remains, they wanted race'.[61] Quite simply, if forensic anthropologists want to retain (and of course enhance, as is the way of the world) their practical aspect they need to read the inscriptions of racial categories on bare decomposed human corpses, not educate the masses that racial categories are not really in the flesh. In this regard, forensic anthropology is forced into a naturalistic biopolitical stand, tracing political categorizations and identities to their alleged biological origins.

In this, forensic anthropologists are in no way unique, since it was the attempt of physicians in the first half of the twentieth century to carve new niches of applied expertise for themselves that fuelled the initial development of naturalistic biopolitics in its organistic version.[62] This said, as discussed above, forensic anthropology has more to it than the willingness to supply society with the allegedly biological underpinnings its discourse of legitimation requires. When working with skeletonized human remains from events of mass violence and genocide, acting as expert witnesses for international tribunals, a more sophisticated approach appears, in which what is reconstructed from the corpses is the 'gaze of the perpetrator'. In other words, instead of a biologization of political categories and identities, forensic anthropology, when working in the context of the requirements of international humanitarian law, aims to reconstruct, from whatever inscriptions it happened to leave on the corpse, the concrete resonance of the biological life system and the political social system in a particular historical moment.

Conclusion

Biopolitics is the historically specific structural coupling of the political social system and the biological life system. This structural coupling, which is always historically specific, is both inscribed on corpses of mass violence and genocide as well as embodied in such corpses.

Given this, the study of corpses of mass violence and genocide has much to gain from a biopolitical perspective. The first part of this chapter briefly sketched the history of the concept, pointed out the theoretical merits of its Foucaulodian configuration, highlighted the three main problems of applying it to the study of genocide and mass violence, and suggested possible ways of overcoming them.

The second part of the chapter tried to substantiate the conclusions of the first part by suggesting certain analytical insights about corpses of mass violence and genocide. Arguably, the correlationist fallacy of Foucauldian biopolitics can be avoided by paying attention to the potent materiality of corpses, which, in the case of mass violence and genocide, means studying the emergent effects of populations of corpses (for example epidemics, but also hideouts). Likewise the 'functionalist' bias of the biopolitical approach to the study of genocide and mass violence should be countered by studying the way Stone's irrational carnivalesque qualities of genocidal events are produced (together with other things) by the very presence of multiple bare corpses and the effects this has on human behaviour. Such behaviour is of course never simply 'universal and natural', but rather variously historically constructed. Hence, as outlined above, one needs to look into the genealogy (i.e. the various genealogies of different cultures and contexts) of corpses as embodiments of death and the political implications and applications of this embodiment.

The chapter then referred to the biopolitical meaning of the rise of forensic anthropology as a professional and authoritative interpreter of corpses as planes of inscription. Arguably, forensic evidence supplements archival material and oral testimonies, and if allowed to introduce its own original input, may revolutionize existing assumptions concerning genocide and mass violence, which are currently profoundly correlationist and state centric.

Notes

1 G. Agamben, *Homo Sacer: Sovereign Power and Bare Life* (Stanford: Stanford University Press, 1998), p. 181.
2 Roberto Esposito mentions in passing the relevance of Niklas Luhmann's work to biopolitics in *Bios: Biopolitics and Philosophy* (Minneapolis: University of Minnesota Press, 2008 – original Italian edition published in 2004), p. 49; see also Christian Borch's comparative-synthetic discussion of Foucault's and Luhmann's analyses of power, 'Systemic power: Foucault, Luhmann and analytic of power', *Acta Sociologica*, 48 (2005), pp. 155–67. An in-depth introduction to contemporary social systems theory is D. B. Lee & A. Brosziewski, *Observing Society: Meaning, Communication and Social Systems* (Amherst: Cambria Press, 2009); see also F. Geyer & J. van der Zouwen (eds), *Sociocybernetics: Complexity, Autopoiesis, and Observation of Social Systems* (London: Greenwood Press, 2001). Introductory works on Niklas Luhmann by Hans-Georg Moeller are: *Luhmann Explained: From Souls to Systems* (Chicago: Open Court, 2006) and *The Radical Luhmann* (New York: Columbia University Press, 2012). Luhmann's opus magnus is *Social Systems* (Stanford: Stanford University Press, 1995 – original German edition 1984).
3 Thomas Lemke in his excellent *Biopolitics: An Advanced Introduction* (New York: New York University Press, 2011) defines biopolitics as a conceptualization, the suggestive power and potency of which stem from the instability and fragility of the border between 'life' and 'politics', which opens up a field of enquiry and critique that tries to account for the relations between and historicity of life and politics, rather than treating them as isolated phenomena (p. 4).
4 For an intellectual history of biopolitics see Esposito, *Bios*, pp. 13–44; and also Lemke, *Biopolitics*, pp. 9–31.
5 Lemke presents a detailed bibliography of the organicist version of naturalist biopolitics in *Biopolitics*.
6 See for example A. Somit & S. A. Peterson, *Darwinism, Dominance, and Democracy: The Biological Bases of Authoritarianism* (Westport: Praeger, 1997).
7 See Lemke's outline and analysis of the politicist configuration of biopolitics in *Biopolitics*, pp. 23–31. The main examples of works within this configuration of biopolitics are: W. T. Anderson, *To Govern Evolution: Further Adventures of the Political Animal* (Boston: Harcourt Brace Jovanovich, 1987); K. Cauthen, *Christian Biopolitics: A Credo and Strategy for the Future* (Nashville: Abingdon, 1971); and D. Gunst, *Biopolitik zwischen Macht und Recht* (Mainz: Hase und Kohler, 1978).
8 M. Foucault, 'The birth of social medicine', in J. Faubion (ed.), *Power: Essential Works of Michel Foucault* (New York: New Press, 2000), vol. 3, p. 137. The systematic elaboration of the concept was done later, in his 1976 series of lectures in the College de France – M. Foucault, *Society Must Be Defended* (New York: Picador, 2003), pp. 239–64, as well in his *History of Sexuality* (New York: Vintage Books, 1980), vol. 1.

9 See Moeller, *Luhmann Explained*, pp. 41–52.
10 M. H. Nadesan, *Governmentality, Biopower and Everyday Life* (London: Routledge, 2008), pp. 7–9.
11 Foucault, *Society Must Be Defended*, pp. 242–3.
12 Ibid., p. 250.
13 See the discussion by Norbert Wiener – the father of cybernetics – on this transformation in 'Newtonian and Bergsonian time', in *Cybernetics: Or Control and Communication in the Animal and the Machine* (Cambridge: MIT Press, 1948), pp. 30–44.
14 See the original presentation of P. H. Wicksteed, *The Common Sense of Political Economy* (London: Macmillan, 1910); the second chapter is also available at www.econlib.org/library/Wicksteed/wkCS2.html#Book I,Ch.2 (accessed 28 November 2013).
15 See A. W. Neal, 'Cutting off the king's head: Foucault's "Society Must Be Defended" and the problem of sovereignty', *Alternatives: Global, Local, Political*, 29:4 (2004), pp. 373–98.
16 Lemke, *Biopolitics*, pp. 40–4; and see Achillle Mbembe's reading of Bataille with regard to death and sovereignty, 'Necropolitics', *Public Culture*, 15:1 (2003), pp. 11–40.
17 L. Chiesa & A. Toscano (eds), *The Italian Difference: Between Nihilism and Biopolitics* (Melbourne: Re-Press, 2009).
18 Agamben, *Homo Sacer*; G. Agamben, *Remnants of Auschwitz: The Witness and the Archive* (New York: Zone Books, 1999); G. Agamben, *Means Without End: Notes on Politics* (Minneapolis: University of Minnesota Press, 2000); see also J. Clemens, N. Heron & A. Murray (eds), *The Work of Giorgio Agamben: Law, Literature, Life* (Edinburgh: Edinburgh University Press, 2008); L. de la Durantaye, *Giorgio Agamben: A Critical Introduction* (Stanford: Stanford University Press, 2009).
19 M. Hardt & A. Negri, *Empire: The New World Order* (Cambridge: Harvard University Press, 2000); M. Hardt & A. Negri, *Multitude: War and Democracy in the Age of Empire* (New York: Penguin, 2004).
20 Esposito, *Bios*; R. Esposito, *Communitas: The Origin and Destiny of Community* (Stanford: Stanford University Press, 2004); R. Esposito, *Immunitas: The Protection and Negation of Life* (London: Polity Press, 2011); see also *Diacritics*, 36:2 (2006) (special issue on Roberto Esposito); T. Campbell, '*Bios*, immunity, life: the thought of Roberto Esposito', *Diacritics*, 36:2 (2006), pp. 2–22.
21 See for example, M. G. E. Kelly, 'International biopolitics: Foucault, globalization and imperialism', *Theoria*, 57:123 (2010), pp. 1–26.
22 See in this regard M. Levine, *Genocide in the Age of the Nation State, Volume 2: The Rise of the West and the Coming of Genocide* (London: I. B. Tauris, 2005).
23 See the work of Nitzan Lebovic in a special issue about philosophy and theory of Fascism, 'The beauty and terror of life: Ludwig Klages, Walter Benjamin, and Alfred Baeumler', *South Central Review*, 23:1 (2006), pp. 23–39.
24 See Vivian Liska's criticism of Agamben's messianism in *Giorgio Agambens leerer Messianismus* (Vienna: Schlebrügge, 2008); and also

Lorenzo Chiesa, 'Giorgio Agamben's Franciscan ontology', *Cosmos and History: The Journal of Natural and Social Philosophy*, 5:1 (2009), pp. 105–16.
25 Lemke, *Biopolitics*, p. 59; he also mentions P. Fitzpatrick, 'These mad abandon'd times', *Economy and Society*, 30:2 (2001), pp. 255–70.
26 See R. Eaglestone, *The Holocaust and the Postmodern* (Oxford: Oxford University Press, 2004); K. Ball, *Disciplining the Holocaust* (New York: SUNY Press, 2008).
27 See Lemke, *Biopolitics*, pp. 58–63.
28 D. A. Moses, 'Genocide and modernity', in Dan Stone (ed.), *The Historiography of Genocide* (London: Palgrave Macmillan, 2008), pp. 156–93; D. A. Moses, 'Modernity and the Holocaust', *Australian Journal of Politics and History*, 43 (1997), pp. 441–5.
29 D. Stone, 'Biopower and modern genocide', in A. D. Moses (ed.), *Empire, Colony, Genocide: Conquest Occupation and Subaltern Resistance in World History* (New York: Berghahn Books, 2008), pp. 162–80.
30 Ibid., p. 164.
31 Foucault, *Society Must Be Defended*, p. 259.
32 C. Gerlach, *Extremely Violent Societies: Mass Violence in the Twentieth Century World* (Cambridge: Cambridge University Press, 2010), pp. 17–122.
33 Q. Meillassoux, *After Finitude: An Essay on the Necessity of Contingency* (London: Continuum, 2008 – original French edition 2006); for discussion of Meillassoux see L. Bryant, N. Srnicek & G. Harman (eds), *The Speculative Turn: Continental Materialism and Realism* (Melbourne: Re-Press, 2011); G. Harman, *Quentin Meillassoux: Philosophy in the Making* (Edinburgh: Edinburgh University Press, 2011).
34 See R. Brassier, *Nihil Unbound* (London: Palgrave Macmillan, 2007), p. 65.
35 See in this regard Gilles Deleuze's monograph about Foucault, *Foucault* (Minneapolis: University of Minnesota Press, 1988).
36 See Brassier's discussion, *Nihil Unbound*, pp. 49–53.
37 J.-P. Satre, *Nausea* (New York: New Directions, 1964).
38 F. Stepputat, 'Governing the dead: an introduction', in F. Stepputat (ed.), *Governing the Dead: Sovereignty and the Politics of Dead Bodies* (Manchester: Manchester University Press, 2014).
39 See J. Fontein, 'The politics of the dead: living heritage, bones and commemoration in Zimbabwe', at www.theasa.org/publications/asaonline/articles/asaonline0102.pdf (accessed 28 November 2013); J. Fontein, 'Between tortured bodies and resurfacing bones: the politics of the dead in Zimbabwe', *Journal of Material Culture*, 15:4 (2010), pp. 423–8; J. Fontein, C. Krmpotich & J. Harries, 'The substance of bones: the emotive materiality and affective presence of human remains', *Journal of Material Culture*, 15:4 (2010), pp. 371–84; J. Fontein & J. Harries, 'Report of the Bones Collective workshop, 4–5 December 2008', at www.san.ed.ac.uk/_data/assets/pdf_file/0013/29110/Final_Report.pdf (accessed 28 November 2013).
40 J. Kristeva, *Powers of Horror* (New York: Columbia University Press,

1982); see also Cecilia Sjoholm's critical interpretation in *Kristeva and the Political* (London: Routledge, 2005), pp. 95–9.
41 Fontein, 'Between tortured bodies'; J. Fontein, 'Shared legacies of the war: spirit mediums and war veterans in southern Zimbabwe', *Journal of Religion in Africa*, 36:2 (2006), pp. 167–99.
42 G. Harman, *Tool-Being: Heidegger and the Metaphysics of Objects* (Chicago: Open Court, 2002).
43 See P. Ariès, *The Hour of Our Death* (New York: Alfred A. Knopf, 1977).
44 See especially G. Bataille, *The Accursed Share* (New York: Zone Books, 1991), vols 2 and 3; and Charles Taylor, *A Secular Age* (Cambridge: Harvard University Press, 2007).
45 In connection with his thesis regarding corpses as both/neither person and/nor object Fontein cites Paul Geary, 'Sacred commodities: the circulation of medieval relics', in A. Appadurai (ed.), *The Social Life of Things* (Cambridge: Cambridge University Press, 1986), pp. 169–91.
46 P. Brown, *The Cult of the Saints: Its Rise and Function in Latin Christianity* (Chicago: University of Chicago Press, 1981).
47 See for example Charles Taylor's discussion on the emergence of this approach to death in Taylor, *A Secular Age*.
48 Fontein, 'The politics of the dead'.
49 See in this regard the suicide of Slobodan Milošević. M. Scharf & B. Schabas, *Slobodan Milošević on Trial* (New York: Continuum, 2002).
50 In fact this is for Meillassoux the very Archimedic point from which one is able to transcend the correlationist stand. See *After Finitude*, location 821, Kindle edition.
51 See for example C. Joyce & E. Stover, *Witnesses from the Grave: The Stories Bones Tell* (New York: Little, Brown, 1991); C. Koff, *The Bone Woman: A Forensic Anthropologist's Search for Truth in the Mass Graves of Rwanda, Bosnia, Croatia and Kosovo* (New York: Random House, 2005); E. Domanska, 'Toward the archeontology of the dead body', *Rethinking History*, 389:403 (2005), pp. 389–413; E. Stover, W. D. Haglund & M. Samuels, 'Exhumation of mass graves in Iraq: considerations for forensic investigations, humanitarian needs, and the demands of justice', *Journal of the American Medical Association*, 290:5 (2003), pp. 663–6; W. D. Haglund, M. Connor & D. D. Scott, 'The archaeology of contemporary mass graves', *Historical Archaeology*, 35:1 (2001), pp. 57–69.
52 With regard to the tension between the forensic search for evidence and the families right of closure see A. Rosenblatt, 'International forensic investigations and the human rights of the dead', *Human Rights Quarterly*, 32:4 (2010), pp. 921–50.
53 See Stepputat's discussion, 'Governing the dead'.
54 See in this regard M. DeLanda, *Philosophy and Simulation: The Emergence of Synthetic Reason* (New York: Continuum, 2011).
55 See with regard to biohazards produced by large concentrations of corpse in events of mass violence and genocide, Y. Schuliar, P. Juel & T. Knudsen, 'Role of forensic pathologists in mass disasters', *Forensic Science Medical Pathology*, 8 (2012), pp. 164–73.

56 With regard to cannibalism vis-à-vis the critical anthropological discourse suggesting the imagery origins of reports on such phenomena, see J. Pottier, 'Rights violations, rumour, and rhetoric: making sense of cannibalism in Mambasa, Ituri (Democratic Republic of Congo)', *Journal of the Royal Anthropological Institute*, 13 (2007), pp. 825–43.
57 See for example D. A. Komar, 'Variables influencing victim selection in genocide', *Journal of Forensic Sciences*, 53:1 (2008), pp. 172–7.
58 See www.physanth.org/association/position-statements/biological-aspects-of-race/?searchterm=race (accessed 28 November 2013).
59 See www.aaanet.org/stmts/racepp.htm (accessed 28 November 2013).
60 A. G. Morris, *Missing and Murdered: A Personal Adventure in Forensic Anthropology* (Cape Town: Zebra Press, 2011), p. 42.
61 C. B. Quintyn, *The Existence or Non-existence of Race: Forensic Anthropology, Population Admixture and the Future of Racial Classification in the US* (Amherst: Teneo Press, 2010), location 47, Kindle edition.
62 See in this regard Robert J. Lifton's classic *The Nazi Doctors: Medical Killing and the Psychology of Genocide* (New York: Basic Books, 2000).

Bibliography

Agamben, G., *Homo Sacer: Sovereign Power and Bare Life* (Stanford: Stanford University Press, 1998)
Agamben, G., *Means Without End: Notes on Politics* (Minneapolis: University of Minnesota Press, 2000)
Agamben, G., *Remnants of Auschwitz: The Witness and the Archive* (New York: Zone Books, 1999)
Anderson, W. T., *To Govern Evolution: Further Adventures of the Political Animal* (Boston: Harcourt Brace Jovanovich, 1987)
Ariès, P., *The Hour of Our Death* (New York: Afred A. Knopf, 1977)
Ball, K., *Disciplining the Holocaust* (New York: SUNY Press, 2008)
Bataille, G., *The Accursed Share* (New York: Zone Books, 1991), vols 2 and 3
Borch, C., 'Systemic power: Foucault, Luhmann and analytic of power', *Acta Sociologica*, 48 (2005), pp. 155–67
Brassier, R., *Nihil Unbound* (London: Palgrave Macmillan, 2007)
Brown, P., *The Cult of the Saints: Its Rise and Function in Latin Christianity* (Chicago: University of Chicago Press, 1981)
Bryant, L., N. Srnicek & G. Harman (eds), *The Speculative Turn: Continental Materialism and Realism* (Melbourne: Re-Press, 2011)
Campbell, T., '*Bios*, immunity, life: the thought of Roberto Esposito', *Diacritics*, 36:2 (2006), pp. 2–22
Cauthen, K., *Christian Biopolitics: A Credo and Strategy for the Future* (Nashville: Abingdon, 1971)
Chiesa, L., 'Giorgio Agamben's Franciscan ontology', *Cosmos and History: The Journal of Natural and Social Philosophy*, 5:1 (2009), pp. 105–16
Chiesa, L. & A. Toscano (eds), *The Italian Difference: Between Nihilism and Biopolitics* (Melbourne: Re-Press, 2009)

Clemens, J., N. Heron & A. Murray (eds), *The Work of Giorgio Agamben: Law, Literature, Life* (Edinburgh: Edinburgh University Press, 2008)
de la Durantaye, L., *Giorgio Agamben: A Critical Introduction* (Stanford: Stanford University Press, 2009)
DeLanda, M., *Philosophy and Simulation: The Emergence of Synthetic Reason* (New York: Continuum, 2011)
Deleuze, G., *Foucault* (Minneapolis: University of Minnesota Press, 1988)
Diacritics 36:2 (2006) (special issue on Roberto Esposito)
Domanska, E., 'Toward the archeontology of the dead body', *Rethinking History*, 389:403 (2005), pp. 389–413
Eaglestone, R., *The Holocaust and the Postmodern* (Oxford: Oxford University Press, 2004)
Esposito, R., *Bios: Biopolitics and Philosophy* (Minneapolis: University of Minnesota Press, 2008 – original Italian edition published in 2004)
Esposito, R., *Communitas: The Origin and Destiny of Community* (Stanford: Stanford University Press, 2004)
Esposito, R., *Immunitas: The Protection and Negation of Life* (London: Polity Press, 2011)
Fitzpatrick, P., 'These mad abandon'd times', *Economy and Society*, 30:2 (2001), pp. 255–70
Fontein, J., 'Between tortured bodies and resurfacing bones: the politics of the dead in Zimbabwe', *Journal of Material Culture*, 15:4 (2012), pp. 423–48
Fontein, J., 'Shared legacies of the war: spirit mediums and war veterans in southern Zimbabwe', *Journal of Religion in Africa*, 36:2 (2006), pp. 167–99
Fontein, J., 'The politics of the dead: living heritage, bones and commemoration in Zimbabwe', at www.theasa.org/publications/asaonline/articles/asaonline0102.pdf
Fontein, J. & J. Harries, 'Report of the Bones Collective workshop, 4–5 December 2008', at www.san.ed.ac.uk/_data/assets/pdf_file/0013/29110/Final_Report.pdf
Fontein, J., C. Krmpotich & J. Harries, 'The substance of bones: the emotive materiality and affective presence of human remains', *Journal of Material Culture*, 15:4 (2010), pp. 371–84
Foucault, M., *History of Sexuality* (New York: Vintage Books, 1980), vol. 1
Foucault, M., *Society Must Be Defended* (New York: Picador, 2003)
Foucault, M., 'The birth of social medicine', in J. Faubion (ed.), *Power: Essential Works of Michel Foucault* (New York: New Press, 2000), vol. 3, pp. 134–56
Geary, P., 'Sacred commodities: the circulation of medieval relics', in A. Appadurai (ed.), *The Social Life of Things* (Cambridge: Cambridge University Press, 1986), pp. 169–91
Gerlach, C., *Extremely Violent Societies: Mass Violence in the Twentieth Century World* (Cambridge: Cambridge University Press, 2010)
Geyer, F. & J. van der Zouwen (eds), *Sociocybernetics: Complexity, Autopoiesis, and Observation of Social Systems* (London: Greenwood Press, 2001)

Gunst, D., *Biopolitik zwischen Macht und Recht* (Mainz: Hase und Kohler Verlag, 1978)
Haglund, W. D., M. Connor & D. D. Scott, 'The archaeology of contemporary mass graves', *Historical Archaeology*, 35: 1 (2001), pp. 57–69
Hardt, M. & A. Negri, *Empire: The New World Order* (Cambridge: Harvard University Press, 2000)
Hardt, M. & A. Negri, *Multitude: War and Democracy in the Age of Empire* (New York: Penguin, 2004)
Harman, G., *Quentin Meillassoux: Philosophy in the Making* (Edinburgh: Edinburgh University Press, 2011)
Harman, G., *Tool-Being: Heidegger and the Metaphysics of Objects* (Chicago: Open Court, 2002)
Joyce, C. & E. Stover, *Witnesses from the Grave: The Stories Bones Tell* (New York: Little, Brown, 1991)
Kelly, M. G. E., 'International biopolitics: Foucault, globalization and imperialism', *Theoria*, 57:123 (2010), pp. 1–26
Koff, C., *The Bone Woman: A Forensic Anthropologist's Search for Truth in the Mass Graves of Rwanda, Bosnia, Croatia and Kosovo* (New York: Random House, 2005)
Komar, D. A., 'Variables influencing victim selection in genocide', *Journal of Forensic Sciences*, 53:1 (2008), pp. 172–7
Kristeva, J., *Powers of Horror* (New York: Columbia University Press, 1982)
Lebovic, N., 'The beauty and terror of life: Ludwig Klages, Walter Benjamin, and Alfred Baeumler', *South Central Review*, 23:1 (2006), pp. 23–39 (special issue on philosophy and theory of Fascism)
Lee, D. B. & A. Brosziewski, *Observing Society: Meaning, Communication and Social Systems* (Amherst: Cambria Press, 2009)
Lemke, T., *Biopolitics: An Advanced Introduction* (New York: New York University Press, 2011)
Levine, M., *Genocide in the Age of the Nation State, Volume 2: The Rise of the West and the Coming of Genocide* (London: I. B. Tauris, 2005)
Lifton, R. J., *The Nazi Doctors: Medical Killing and the Psychology of Genocide* (New York: Basic Books, 2000)
Liska, V., *Giorgio Agambens leerer Messianismus* (Vienna: Schlebrügge, 2008)
Luhmann, N., *Social Systems* (Stanford: Stanford University Press, 1995 – original German edition 1984)
Mbembe, A., 'Necropolitics', *Public Culture*, 15:1 (2003), pp. 11–40
Meillassoux, Q., *After Finitude: An Essay on the Necessity of Contingency* (London: Continuum, 2008 – original French edition 2006)
Moeller, H.-G., *Luhmann Explained: From Souls to Systems* (Chicago: Open Court, 2006)
Moeller, H.-G., *The Radical Luhmann* (New York: Columbia University Press, 2012)
Morris, A. G., *Missing and Murdered: A Personal Adventure in Forensic Anthropology* (Cape Town: Zebra Press, 2011)
Moses, D. A., 'Genocide and modernity', in D. Stone (ed.), *The Historiography of Genocide* (London: Palgrave Macmillan, 2008), pp. 156–93

Moses, D. A., 'Modernity and the Holocaust', *Australian Journal of Politics and History*, 43 (1997), pp. 441–5

Nadesan, M. H., *Governmentality, Biopower and Everyday Life* (London: Routledge, 2008)

Neal, A. W., 'Cutting off the king's head: Foucault's "Society Must Be Defended" and the problem of sovereignty', *Alternatives: Global, Local, Political*, 29:4 (2004), pp. 373–98

Pottier, J., 'Rights violations, rumour, and rhetoric: making sense of cannibalism in Mambasa, Ituri (Democratic Republic of Congo)', *Journal of the Royal Anthropological Institute*, 13 (2007), pp. 825–43

Quintyn, C. B., *The Existence or Non-existence of Race: Forensic Anthropology, Population Admixture and the Future of Racial Classification in the US* (Amherst: Teneo Press, 2010)

Rosenblatt, A., 'International forensic investigations and the human rights of the dead', *Human Rights Quarterly*, 32:4 (2010), pp. 921–50

Sartre, J.-P., *Nausea* (New York: New Directions, 1964)

Scharf, M. & B. Schabas, *Slobodan Milošević on Trial* (New York: Continuum, 2002)

Schuliar, Y., P. Juel & T. Knudsen, 'Role of forensic pathologists in mass disasters', *Forensic Science Medical Pathology*, 8 (2012), pp. 164–73

Sjoholm, C., *Kristeva and the Political* (London: Routledge, 2005)

Somit, A. & S. A. Peterson, *Darwinism, Dominance, and Democracy: The Biological Bases of Authoritarianism* (Westport: Praeger, 1997)

Stepputat, F., 'Governing the dead.: an introduction', in F. Stepputat (ed.), *Governing the Dead: Sovereignty and the Politics of Dead Bodies* (Manchester: Manchester University Press, 2014)

Stone, D., 'Biopower and modern genocide', in A. D. Moses (ed.), *Empire, Colony, Genocide: Conquest Occupation and Subaltern Resistance in World History* (New York: Berghahn Books, 2008), pp. 162–80

Stover, E., W. D. Haglund & M. Samuels, 'Exhumation of mass graves in Iraq: considerations for forensic investigations, humanitarian needs, and the demands of justice', *Journal of the American Medical Association*, 290:5 (2003), pp. 663–6

Taylor, C., *A Secular Age* (Cambridge: Harvard University Press, 2007)

Wicksteed, P. H., *The Common Sense of Political Economy* (London: Macmillan, 1910)

Wiener, N., 'Newtonian and Bergsonian time', in *Cybernetics: Or Control and Communication in the Animal and the Machine* (Cambridge: Massachusetts Institute of Technology Press, 1948), pp. 30–44

2

Seeking the dead among the living: embodying the disappeared of the Argentinian dictatorship through law[1]

Sévane Garibian

> Y así seguimos andando
> curtidos de soledad,
> y en nosotros nuestros muertos
> pa' que nadie quede atrás.
> (Atahualpa Yupanqui[2])

Introduction

The state policy of enforced disappearances in Argentina, planned and implemented during the military dictatorship of 1976–83, still has a striking effect today: in the absence of any corpses of the disappeared, the families *seek the dead among the living*. Their quest through the law *embodies* the victims who were 'disappeared' and thereby placed *outside of the law*: 'we might say that the absolutely defeated person is the outlaw, the disappeared. This was indeed [Walter] Benjamin's thesis on the vanquished of history: those who leave no traces, those whose bodies cannot be shown, any more than the story of their end, have deserved their fate: to have none.'[3] From this perspective, disappearance is a challenge to the law.[4]

To find a juridical solution to the enigma of disappearance is to treat the disappeared precisely as *disappeared*, not as deceased, through the law, from which, in the executioner's point of view, the disappeared is excluded, as non-existent. Even the former head of the military junta, Jorge Videla, said in a confession recently collected and published by the Argentinian journalist Ceferino Reato that 'every disappearance might be understood as a masking, a concealment of death'.[5] We find the echo of this substantive denial in the international definition of the crime of enforced disappearance, which includes a 'refusal to acknowledge the deprivation of liberty or concealment of the fate or whereabouts of the disappeared person, which places such a person outside the protection of the law'.[6]

Moreover, still from the juridical perspective, this substantive denial makes enforced disappearance a *continuous crime*,[7] thus creating an interesting paradox: so long as the disappeared body is not found, the crime of disappearance (denied by the executioner – 'there are no disappeared, but absentees who will return'[8]) continues while at the same time being deprived of its physical, material and 'corporeal' proof. In other words, the crime of disappearance continues as long as the *corpus delicti* is not provided, or as long as its history is not retraced: the crime is perpetuated by its own effacement, through its effect on the families of the victims and, more generally, within a society weary of the activist injunction, the cry, the tirelessly reiterated slogan 'Present! Now and forever' (*¡Presente ahora y para siempre!*).[9] This is the locus of the 'infamy of the disappearance': 'indefinitely prolonged doubt, for the disappearance is an event that lasts forever. What lasts forever is that a person I can name is neither present nor absent.... The disappeared "is" in the middle of neither, nor.'[10]

It is thus a question of reversal: if the nature of war is to turn the corpse of the Other ('the enemy without') into a trophy and a proof of victory, then, conversely, the nature of the policy of enforced disappearance is to turn the corpse of the Self ('the enemy within') into an absence, a non-fact, a *neither–nor* – a double negative that strangely recalls the NN of *Nomen nescio*[11] or the Hitlerian *Nacht und Nebel* (Night and Fog) directive.[12] According to Lefeuvre-Déotte, 'The technique of disappearance not only attacks the life of a supposed enemy, it robs it of death, dissolves, and pulverizes it. It aims to destroy this essential human dichotomy, of life and death, creating a special category, that of neither living nor dead.'[13] The body of the disappeared – 'sucked up' (*chupado*) as it was previously termed in Argentinian military jargon[14] – then becomes the missing evidence of the crime. Moreover, and most interestingly, 'not seeing the corpse reinforces denial of the death',[15] which is entirely crystallized in the slogan of some of the mothers of the Plaza de Mayo when they claim maternity has been reversed (the disappeared children have given birth to them and they – the mothers – are born into the struggle) and the disappeared appear again alive (¡Aparición con vida!).[16]

Within this entirely unusual configuration of mass state violence constructed on the systematic effacement of the bodies of its victims, we shall attempt to comprehend the disappeared body as the object of a triple challenge: establishment of the facts, to bring them into the light, the (re)construction and understanding of the narrative of what took place; the exposure of the crime and sentencing of those responsible; and an end to the crime and access to mourning. It then becomes a question of thinking of the disappeared/absent body not 'in the negative', in respect of what it prevents, but 'in the positive', in respect of what it allows juridically: that is, to think of it as generating rights and duties. The absence of the bodies of the disappeared and the demands of the families of the victims in the face of such absence are in fact at the origin of the unusual creation of a new human right in Argentina: the right to the truth (*derecho a la verdad*). Recognition of this new subjective right (protecting the families and relatives of the victims) is mirrored by recognition of the state's duty to vigorously investigate the very body, present or alive, of the 'stolen children' of the dictatorship, in the search for the identity and the fate of them all. The *derecho a la verdad* thus becomes the key to understanding the implementation of two kinds of extraordinary procedures, quite specific to the Argentinian case, that *give body* to the disappeared through the law. The first is direct: the sanctionless so-called 'truth hearings' for the reconstruction of their fate. The second is indirect, by means of procedures for the mandatory recovery of the identity of their stolen children. Both actually constitute antechambers of the classic penal process for the trial of those accused of carrying out enforced disappearances and stealing the children of the disappeared (abducted at the same time as their parents, as discussed in the last section of the chapter). If the disappearance is, initially, a challenge to the law, the law thus becomes, in turn, a challenge to the disappearance.

Right to the truth and reconstruction of the fate of the disappeared

Argentina is an extraordinary laboratory in the domain of struggle against impunity and of 'restoration of the truth', and constitutes a useful paradigm in the context of reflection on the corpses of mass violence. Its special character, in the immediate aftermath of the military dictatorship, is to test almost the entirety of juridical mechanisms in the handling of state crimes: adoption of self-amnesty under the military government of General Reynaldo Bignone, in the name of 'pacification of the country' and of 'social reconciliation' just before his fall; then the creation of the National Commission on the Disappearance of Persons (Comisión Nacional sobre la Desaparición de Personas, CONADEP) by Raúl Alfonsín, initiator of the democratic transition (1983); the publication in 1984 of the famous report *Nunca más* (*Never Again*) on the Commission's work; then the organization in 1985 of the trial of the generals in the first three military juntas; a further promulgation of two amnesties by the same Alfonsín (1986–87); the signature of reprieves (*indultos*) and presidential pardon granted in 1990 by Carlos Menem to all the condemned of the 1985 trial; parliamentary annulment of the amnesty laws after the election of Nestor Kirchner in 2003; followed by the declaration of their unconstitutionality by the Supreme Court in 2005 and the reopening of criminal prosecutions.[17]

Within the critical period between the adoption of the amnesty laws of 1986–87 and their recent annulment, there emerged and became established the *derecho a la verdad* associated with an alternative judicial practice, *sui generis* and unique in the world: the sanctionless truth hearing (*juicios por la verdad*), a genuine national singularity that was confected in reaction to the policy of forgetting the 1990s and of the blocking of criminal prosecutions until 2005. It all began on 3 March 1995, when the former naval captain Adolfo Scilingo made a public admission of his active participation in the 'death flights' for the first time.[18] This sent an electric shock through Argentinian civil society and marked the start of new claims by the families of the disappeared, demanding resumption of investigations by the state to discover the fate of the victims.

The main aim of the families then was to counter the juridical lock maintained by the amnesty laws still in force at the time, by launching a new kind of action for the right to the truth – just emerging from the (very committed) jurisprudence of the Inter-American Court of Human Rights,[19] but as yet undefined and, moreover, absent from Argentinian law. The national context of this period is even more interesting and richer than in 1994, when a profound reform of the Argentinian constitution was made in a spirit of post-dictatorship 'democratic consolidation'.[20] The latter enabled the principal international instruments for the protection of human rights to be integrated into the Argentinian juridical order, giving them, in addition, a constitutional value in the normative hierarchy.[21]

Between truth commission and classic criminal prosecution, between symbolic reparation and retribution, the hybrid practice of the *juicios por la verdad* offers a new approach in the judges' mission, no longer punitive but simply *declarative*. What this particular framework demands is not the judgement and criminal conviction of persons charged with serious violations of human rights, but knowledge of the fate of victims by disclosure and clarification of the facts (including the search for and identification of the corpses), combined with judicial recognition of the factual truth, beyond the binary dialectic of guilty/not guilty.

After many twists and turns, the Inter-American Commission on Human Rights reached a friendly agreement, signed on 15 November 1999, under which the Argentinian government would recognize and guarantee the right to the truth, specifying that this right assumed the implementation of all possible means for 'clarification' (*esclarecimiento*) of the fate of the disappeared. This event is totally decisive. It allows for the systematization of the truth hearing in Argentina, in particular before the Federal Chamber in La Plata, where more than 2,000 disappearances were later the subject of public sessions every Wednesday.[22]

At Argentina's further initiative, the United Nations Commission on Human Rights adopted on 20 April 2005 the first resolution on the right to the truth. Argentina is one of the states that worked hardest for the adoption of the International Convention for the Protection of All Persons from Enforced Disappearance, in 2006,[23] which enshrines the right of each relative to know the truth regarding the circumstances of the enforced disappearance, the progress and results of the investigation, and the fate of the disappeared person.[24] In April 2008, Argentina made a commitment before the United Nations Human Rights Council to prepare an international declaration on the right to the truth and memory, as a step towards subsequent drafting of a universal treaty on the subject. This development in the international and United Nations community led on 21 December 2010 to the proclamation by the United Nations General Assembly of 24 March as 'International Day for the Right to the Truth Concerning Gross Human Rights Violations and for the Dignity of Victims'. Parallel with this juridical development, the guarantee of the right to the truth also became an important issue in the context of a new series of cases:

those concerning the mandatory recovery of the children stolen during the dictatorship period.

Right to the truth and mandatory recovery of the identity of stolen children

The systematic practice of enforced disappearances also involved the stealing of an estimated 500 children of the disappeared – children abducted at the same time as their parents, or born in captivity, then stolen as 'spoils of war' (*botín de guerra*) by the soldiers.[25] Later they were given either to members of the armed forces or to civilians, or were legally adopted by families sometimes unaware of their origin (in most cases, the judicial authority approving the adoption had – by contrast – knowledge of the precise facts). At the time of writing, 105 stolen children had been 'restored' after recovery of their lost identity. Among them, ten children had had to undergo a state-enforced recovery of their identity by being DNA tested against their will.[26] These ten cases at the heart of the procedures are our concern here.

The cases in question began at the start of the 2000s: what was at stake was to determine – and on what basis – it would be juridically possible to impose DNA tests on non-consenting persons who were presumed to be stolen children. The special feature of these cases is that they oppose two types of victims of the dictatorship, recognized as such both by the doctrine and by the jurisprudence (national and inter-American) of human rights: the families of the disappeared and their stolen children, who bear in them the traces of their disappeared parents – 'there is always a *remnant* in the person of the surviving witness'.[27]

Two main rights were then in conflict, which the judges had to consider: on the one hand, the right to the truth invoked by families seeking the bodies of the disappeared and the identity of their stolen children; on the other, the right to privacy claimed by some of these children who refused to undergo DNA tests, either voluntarily (from loyalty to their adoptive parents), or not (under pressure or threat from the latter). The right to the truth is most often invoked in association with the right to protection of family relations, the right to reparation for the stealing of children by the state, or the right to personal integrity. As for the right to privacy, it is claimed together with its primary corollaries (the right to self-determination, the right to free choice of a life plan and the right not to know one's biological identity) and/or its secondary corollaries (the right not to testify against one's parents or kin, the right to bodily integrity and the right to mental health).

Argentina's Supreme Court, from 2003, ruled several times on this question of the balance between the right to the truth and the right to privacy.[28] In respect of minors, the Court's tendency has always been to approve the imposition of DNA tests, on the principle of 'the child's best interest', the right to privacy and the duty of the state to prosecute those responsible for the stealing of children. In respect of adults, the jurisprudence is evolving. Since 2009 the Court has regarded the right to the truth (directly associated with the state's duty to investigate and prosecute serious violations of human rights) as more important than the right to privacy. In other words, in the Court's opinion, the latter cannot constitute an obstacle to the recovery of the identity of stolen children, and the right to the truth justifies the state 'going into the body' (*ponerse en el cuerpo*) by force, if that is necessary for carrying out its duties, and if the sampling methods ordered by a judge for a test are reasonable, proportionate and appropriate to the circumstances and the desired goal.

The right to privacy capitulates to the right to truth – the latter being understood as an absolute right that therefore legitimizes state interference in the human being whose body, moreover, becomes a potential piece of evidence in the policy of enforced disappearances. This legal jurisdictional interpretation is enshrined in a new article of the criminal procedure code (article 218 bis), into which it was incorporated in 2009, following a friendly agreement between the Argentinian state and the Inter-American Commission on Human Rights.[29] The regulation further clarifies that the rules limiting witness testimony against parents or kin and the right to abstain on the matter (articles 242 and 243 of the code) do not apply in this case.

However questionable this now legalized state interference may be, it is no less true that the carrying out of DNA tests regardless of the will or consent of the presumed stolen children has one benefit: that of easing the guilt arising from a conflict of loyalty towards their adoptive parents, or the fear provoked by threats and pressures. And all of this – these feelings of guilt and fear – occur in an already highly charged context where, in most cases, their previously unknown true origins are brutally revealed. Moreover, there is a kind of ricochet: the truth of the role played by the adoptive family in the disappearance of their own biological parents and/or their complicity in state terrorism. On the other hand, the current juridical procedures also avoid the need to make these children responsible for the criminal conviction (or, alternatively, for the impunity) of their adoptive parents, while respecting the public character of the penal process. Paradoxically, the 'duty' of state interference in the matter may be seen above all as a way to confront the state with its own responsibility.

In short, the guarantee of the right of the victims' relatives to the truth – initially created to cover a *gap* – is systematically understood by the judges as inseparable from the dual international state duty of investigating and prosecuting massive violations of human rights. The first state duty is precisely expressed in the truth hearings and the procedures for mandatory recovery of the identity of stolen children. The second duty is expressed in parallel in the classic criminal trials of those responsible for the disappearances and the stealing of the children of the disappeared – 'the latter being required so that the parents of the disappeared detainees might "have" the bodies, to "produce" before the courts'.[30]

All these legal processes, then, are a means of bringing an ongoing crime to an end and according judicial recognition to victims and their families. By embodying the disappeared of the dictatorship, these processes free the bodies of the living.

Notes

1 The text of this chapter was translated from the author's French by Cadenza Academic Translations.
2 Extract from the song 'Los Hermanos' by Héctor Roberto Chavero, also known as Atahualpa Yupanqui, Argentinian poet, singer and guitarist: 'And so we keep wandering / hardened to solitude, / and our dead within us / so as to leave no one behind'. Translations here and below by the translator.
3 'On peut dire alors que le vaincu absolu, c'est le hors-la-loi: le disparu. C'était bien là la thèse de Benjamin concernant les vaincus de l'histoire: ceux qui n'ont pas laissé de traces. Ceux-là dont les cadavres ne peuvent être exposés, pas plus que l'histoire de leur fin, ont bien mérité leur sort: ne pas en avoir.' J.-L. Déotte, 'Les paradoxes de l'événement d'une disparition', in C. Coquio (ed.), *L'Histoire trouée: négation et témoignage* (Nantes: L'Atalante, 2003), p. 557.
4 See also M. Nichanian, 'Le droit et le fait: la campagne de 1994', *Lignes*, 26 (October 1995), p. 88.
5 'Cada desaparición puede ser entendida como el enmascaramiento, el disimulo de una muerte'. Extract from C. Reato, *Disposición final*:

la confesión de Videla sobre los desaparecidos (Buenos Aires: Editorial Sudamericana, 2012).

6 'le déni de la reconnaissance de la privation de liberté ou de la dissimulation du sort réservé à la personne disparue…, la soustrayant à la protection de la loi'. Article 2 of the International Convention for the Protection of All Persons from Enforced Disappearance (adopted 20 December 2006).

7 See article 8, para. 1(b), of the 2006 Convention. The statute of limitations of the crime commences from the moment the offence of enforced disappearance ceases, taking into account its continuous nature.

8 'il n'y a pas de disparus, mais des absents qui reviendront'. Déotte, 'Les paradoxes de l'événement', p. 557.

9 This slogan was taken up by almost all the non-governmental organizations (NGOs) and associations of families of the disappeared in Argentina, and is and was often used in the annual commemorative demonstrations of 24 March (24 March 1976 being the date of the military coup d'état).

10 'infamie de la disparition': 'un doute indéfiniment prolongé, car la disparition est un événement qui dure toujours.… Ce qui dure toujours, c'est qu'une personne que je peux nommer n'est ni présente ni absente. […] Le disparu "est" au milieu du ni, ni'. Déotte, 'Les paradoxes de l'événement', pp. 557–8.

11 Literally 'I do not know the name'. This Latin expression is used to designate an anonymous or undefined person.

12 *Nacht und Nebel* (Night and Fog) was the codename of the operation based on a decree of 7 December 1941 that provided for the arrest of any person representing 'a danger to the security of the German Army', and for the transfer of that person to Germany for eventual disappearance in absolute secrecy.

13 'La technique de la disparition ne s'attaque pas seulement à la vie d'un ennemi supposé, elle lui ôte même sa mort, la dissout et la pulvérise.… Elle cherche à détruire cette distinction essentielle pour l'espèce humaine: celle de la vie et de la mort, en instituant une catégorie particulière, celle du ni vivant, ni mort'. M. Lefeuvre-Déotte, 'La mort dissoute. Un cas: l'Argentine', *Quasimodo*, 9 (2006), p. 99.

14 See for example the witness statement of the survivor P. Calveiro, 'La mémoire comme virus. Pouvoir concentrationnaire et disparition de personnes en Argentine', in C. Coquio (ed.), *L'Histoire trouée: négation et témoignage* (Nantes: L'Atalante, 2003), p. 541.

15 'ne pas voir le cadavre conforte "follement" le déni de la mort'. Lefeuvre-Déotte, 'La mort dissoute'.

16 After 1985, the association Mothers of the Plaza de Mayo split in two: on one side, the movement led by Hebe de Bonafini, which persists in a radical demand for the appearance alive of their disappeared children – 'Con vida los llevaron, con vida los queremos' ('Alive they took them, alive we want them); on the other, the 'founding line', one of whose spokeswomen is Laura Bonaparte, which supports a different approach and supports the search for and identification of the bodies.

17 For an overview see S. Lefranc, 'L'Argentine contre ses généraux: un charivari judiciaire?', *Critique Internationale*, 26 (January 2005), pp. 23–34.
18 The death flights were a practice systematized during the dictatorship, in which thousands of the disappeared were drugged and thrown alive from military aircraft into the Rio de la Plata. The confession, collected by the Argentinian journalist Horacio Verbitsky, was published in English as H. Verbitsky, *The Flight: Confessions of an Argentine Dirty Warrior* (trans. E. Allen) (New York: New Press, 1996), from the Spanish, H. Verbitsky, *El Vuelo: la guerre sale en Argentina* (Buenos Aires: Planeta, 1995).
19 See E. Lambert Abdelgawad & K. Martin-Chenut (eds), *Réparer les violations graves et massives des droits de l'homme: la Cour interaméricaine, pionnière et modèle?* (Paris: Société de législation comparée, 2010).
20 J.-M. Blanquer, 'Consolidation démocratique? Pour une approche constitutionnelle', *Pouvoirs: L'Amérique Latine*, 98 (2001), pp. 37–47.
21 Through the instrument of the new article 75, para. 22, of the constitution. For developments, see H. Tigroudja, 'Le droit international dans les états d'Amérique latine: regards sur l'ordre juridique argentin', *Revue Internationale de Droit Comparé*, 1 (2008), pp. 89–119.
22 See the website of Asemblea permanente por los derechos humanos La Plata (APDH), at http://apdhlaplata.org.ar/v1/category/juicio-por-la-verdad (accessed 20 March 2013). For a detailed study on the right to the truth and the new judicial mechanism of truth hearings, see S. Garibian, 'Derecho a la verdad. El caso argentino', in S. R. Carulla & C. V. Duran (eds), *Justicia de transición: el caso de España* (Barcelona: International Catalan Institute for Peace (ICIP), 2012), pp. 51–63 (accessible in digital format on www.gencat.cat/icip, accessed 9 January 2014), and S. Garibian, 'Vérité vs. impunité. La justice (post-)transitionnelle en Argentine et le *human rights turn*', in K. Andrieu & G. Lauvau (eds), *Quelle justice pour les peuples en transition? Pacifier, démocratiser, réconcilier* (Paris: Presses Universitaires de Paris-Sorbonne, 2014), pp. 287–305. See also S. Garibian, 'Les procès de mémoire sont justifiés: créer de nouveaux outils juridiques', *Le Monde*, 15 April 2011, p. 19.
23 Argentina was also one of the first countries to have ratified that Convention, on 14 December 2007.
24 Preamble and article 24, para. 2, of the 2006 Convention.
25 For complete and updated information, see the website of the association Abuelas de Plaza de Mayo (Grandmothers of the Plaza de Mayo) charged with the search for the stolen (grand)children, at www.abuelas.org.ar (accessed 20 March 2013).
26 We should remember that 1987 was the year when, at the initiative of the grandmothers, a national genetic databank was officially created for the identification of the disappeared and, where appropriate, their stolen children. Scientific advances resulting in the practice of DNA testing then revolutionized the searches and the judicial use of their results in the context of trials.

27 'il y a toujours un *reste* en la personne du témoin survivant'. C. Coquio, 'À propos d'un nihilisme contemporain: négation, déni, témoignage', in C. Coquio (ed.), *L'Histoire trouée: négation et témoignage* (Nantes: L'Atalante, 2003), p. 34.
28 For a detailed analysis of this jurisprudence, see N. Piñol Sala, 'La obligación del estado de restituir la identidad a las víctimas de desaparición forzada', in *Jurisprudencia de la Corte Suprema de Justicia de la Nación* (Buenos Aires: Hammurabi, 2010), vol. 8, p. 312; and J. G. Bongiovanni Servera & J. Gabriel, *La prueba de ADN en el proceso penal: análisis del artículo 218 bis del Código Procesal Penal de la Nación y su discusión parlamentaria* (Buenos Aires: Editores del Puerto, 2012); and A. Iud, 'La apropiación de niños y el análisis de ADN obligatorio', in G. I. Anitua & M. Gaitan (eds), *Las pruebas genéticas en la identificación de jóvenes desaparecidos* (Buenos Aires: Editores Del Puerto, 2012).
29 On this reform, see L. Filippini & K. Terrina, 'ADN: el nuevo art. 218, CPPN', *Revista de Derecho Penal y Procesal Penal* (May 2010), pp. 842-7.
30 'il s'agissait bien de cela, pour les parents des détenus disparus: "avoir" les corps, [les] "produire" devant la justice'. G. E. Mango, *La Place des mères* (Paris: Gallimard, 1999), p. 18.

Bibliography

Blanquer, J.-M., 'Consolidation démocratique? Pour une approche constitutionnelle', *Pouvoirs: L'Amérique Latine*, 98 (2001), pp. 37-47
Bongiovanni Servera, J. G. & J. Gabriel, *La prueba de ADN en el proceso penal. Análisis del artículo 218 bis del Código Procesal Penal de la Nación y su discusión parlamentaria* (Buenos Aires: Editores del Puerto, 2012)
Calveiro, P., 'La mémoire comme virus. Pouvoir concentrationnaire et disparition de personnes en Argentine', in C. Coquio (ed.), *L'Histoire trouée: négation et témoignage* (Nantes: L'Atalante, 2003), pp. 537-56
Coquio, C., 'A propos d'un nihilisme contemporain: négation, déni, témoignage', in C. Coquio (ed.), *L'Histoire trouée: négation et témoignage* (Nantes: L'Atalante, 2003), pp. 23-89
Déotte, J.-L., 'Les paradoxes de l'événement d'une disparition', in C. Coquio (ed.), *L'Histoire trouée: négation et témoignage* (Nantes: L'Atalante, 2003)
Filippini, L. & K. Therian, 'ADN: el nuevo art. 218, CPPN', *Revista de Derecho Pernal y Procesal Penal* (May 2010), pp. 842-7
Garibian, S., 'Derecho a la verdad. El caso argentino', in S. R. Carulla & C. V. Duran (eds), *Justicia de transición: el caso de España* (Barcelona: International Catalan Institute for Peace (ICIP), 2012), pp. 51-63
Garibian, S., 'Les procès de mémoire sont justifiés: créer de nouveaux outils juridiques', *Le Monde*, 15 April 2011, p. 19
Garibian, S., 'Vérité *vs.* impunité. La justice (post-)transitionnelle en Argentine et le *human rights turn*', in K. Andrieu & G. Lauvau (eds), *Quelle*

justice pour les peuples en transition? Pacifier, démocratiser, réconcilier (Paris: Presses Universitaires de la Sorbonne, 2014), pp. 287–305.

Iud, A., 'La apropiación de niños y el análisis de ADN obligatorio', in G. I. Anitua & M. Gaitan (eds), *Las pruebas genéticas en la identificación de jóvenes desaparecidos* (Buenos Aires: Editions Del Puerto, 2012)

Lambert Abdelgawad, E. & K. Martin-Chenut (eds), *Réparer les violations graves et massives des droits de l'homme: la Cour interaméricaine, pionnière et modèle?* (Paris: Société de Législation Comparée, 2010)

Lefeuvre-Déotte, M., 'La mort dissoute. Un cas: l'Argentine', *Quasimodo*, 9 (2006), p. 99

Lefranc, S., 'L'Argentine contre ses généraux: un charivari judiciaire?', *Critique Internationale*, 26 (January 2005), pp. 23–34

Mango, G. E., *La Place des mères* (Paris: Editions Gallimard, 1999)

Nichanian, M., 'Le droit et le fait: la campagne de 1994', *Lignes*, 26 (October 1995), p. 88

Piñol Sala N., 'La obligación del estado de restituir la identidad a las víctimas de desaparición forzada', in *Jurisprudencia de la Corte Suprema de Justicia de la Nación* (Buenos Aires: Hammurabi, 2010), vol. 8

Reato, C., *Disposición final: la confesión de Videla sobre los desaparecidos* (Buenos Aires: Editorial Sudamericana, 2012)

Tigroudja, H., 'Le droit international dans les *états* d'Amérique latine: regards sur l'ordre juridique argentin', *Revue Internationale de Droit Comparé*, 1 (2008), pp. 89–119

Verbitsky, H., *El Vuelo: la guerre sale en Argentina* (Buenos Aires: Planeta, 1995)

Verbitsky, H., *The Flight: Confessions of an Argentine Dirty Warrior* (trans. E. Allen) (New York: New Press, 1996)

Websites

Abuelas de Plaza de Mayo, city of Buenos Aires, at www.abuelas.org.ar

Asemblea permanente por los derechos humanos (APDH), city of La Plata, at http://apdhlaplata.org.ar/v1/category/juicio-por-la-verdad

3

The human body: victim, witness and evidence of mass violence[1]

Caroline Fournet

Introduction

In the context of international criminal law and case law, the fact that the individual, as a human being, is the target of criminals against humanity and *génocidaires* alike is a legal reality that raises no doubt or controversy.[2] The definition of a crime against humanity protects 'any civilian population',[3] while that of genocide refers to the victim 'group'.[4] Further, both definitions protect the physical and moral integrity of the individual – although the text of the law generally refrains from using the word 'body', a reluctance which, as it will be further developed, is not shared by the International Criminal Tribunals or by the International Criminal Court (ICC).

The individual, the first beneficiary of international criminal law, is thus protected in terms of his/her physical and moral integrity, to adopt the terminology used in the legal definitions of crimes of mass violence, or in his/her body and dignity, to refer to the case law of the International Criminal Tribunal for Rwanda (ICTR) and that for the former Yugoslavia (ICTY), as well as of the ICC. This semantic divergence, however slight it might seem, is not devoid of legal consequences at the normative, definitional and procedural level. The present analysis explores this linguistic impact on the judicial understanding of crimes of mass violence and their punishment by international bodies. The International Criminal Tribunals and the ICC generally avoid exercises in style and language of a literary purport. As will be developed, the choice of words here is not without import and the recurring use in their decisions and judgments of the word 'body', although missing from the legal norm, has admittedly paved the way for a more acute comprehension of mass violence. And indeed, the main issue with the text of international criminal law is not so much its cautiousness in using the word 'body', and its preference for the expression 'physical integrity', as its omission of the consideration of the fate inflicted on the human body in the context of mass violence. If 'physical integrity' and 'body' reflect the same reality, the legal norm does not go much further in the perception of the human body, thus neglecting both the significance of the body in the criminal modus operandi and its evidentiary value. This lacuna has not escaped the attention of the international criminal institutions and, as this chapter will demonstrate, by means of a discreet semantic shift, the 'body' and the 'corpse'[5] have entered the legal scene through the judicial door, enabling judges not only to better grasp the very nature of mass violence, as crimes consciously attacking the bodies of victims (the subject of the first section of this chapter), but also to adequately adjudicate such crimes based on the proof provided by the treatment inflicted by criminals on the bodies of their victims (in the second section).

The human body, outward covering of human dignity

> In the death threat, which I felt for the first time in full clarity while reading the laws of Nuremberg, there also lay what is commonly referred to as the methodical 'degradation' of the Jews by the Nazis. Put differently: in the denial of human dignity itself sounded the death threat.[6]

Although it underlies the very phrase 'crime against humanity', human dignity remains a rather elusive concept, since international criminal law refrains from defining it. The contemporary definition of crimes against humanity, as enshrined in the 1998 Rome Statute of the International Criminal Court – whose extended list of prohibited acts is to be applauded – mentions neither human dignity nor the human body as such. The Rome Statute recognizes the following as crimes against humanity:

(a) Murder;
(b) Extermination;
(c) Enslavement;

(d) Deportation or forcible transfer of population;
(e) Imprisonment or other severe deprivation of physical liberty in violation of fundamental rules of international law;
(f) Torture;
(g) Rape, sexual slavery, enforced prostitution, forced pregnancy, enforced sterilization, or any other form of sexual violence of comparable gravity;
(h) Persecution against any identifiable group or collectivity on political, racial, national, ethnic, cultural, religious, gender as defined in paragraph 3, or other grounds that are universally recognized as impermissible under international law, in connection with any act referred to in this paragraph or any crime within the jurisdiction of the Court;
(i) Enforced disappearance of persons;
(j) The crime of apartheid;
(k) Other inhumane acts of a similar character intentionally causing great suffering, or serious injury to body or to mental or physical health.[7]

An explicit reference to the 'human body' within this definition might seem purely rhetorical since the text of the law does protect the physical integrity of the human being (since 'physical integrity' expressly refers to the human body, there is strictly no doubt that the human body as such is protected by the prohibition of 'serious injury to body or to mental or physical health').[8] The document 'Elements of Crimes' (under the Rome Statute) also specifies that prohibited inhumane acts encompass 'great suffering' and 'serious injury to *body* or to mental or physical health'.[9] Even if only implicitly, the human body is likewise protected by the prohibition of torture, in the context of which '[t]he perpetrator inflicted severe physical or mental pain or suffering upon one or more persons',[10] by that of forced pregnancy, as '[t]he perpetrator confined one or more women forcibly made pregnant',[11] and that of forced sterilization, which deprives the victim of '*biological* reproductive capacity'.[12]

Is it this inescapable link between physical integrity and the human body that has prompted the judges of the International Criminal Tribunals to be more explicit and to take an express interest in the human body? Are the judges aware of their interpretation or is it a matter of involuntary – or unreflective – use of the word 'body'? If this chapter does not pretend to provide a definitive answer to these questions, it is nonetheless true that the very expression 'human body', missing from the text of the law – at least in its French version – has incontestably been integrated into the judicial language relative to crimes against humanity.

It is, in this respect, particularly striking that the human body is not mentioned with regard to the crime against humanity of murder – no more than a simple specification that '[t]he perpetrator killed one or more persons'[13] – nor with regard to that of extermination – in which context '[t]he conduct constituted, or took place as part of, a mass killing of members of a civilian population'.[14] This legislative lacuna, however, has not prevented the ICTR Trial Chamber, in its *Akayesu* decision, from proceeding to a meticulous analysis of the murders perpetrated, which includes numerous references to the human body – with a preference in the original English version of the judgment for the word 'body' rather than 'corpse'.[15] Yet, it would be premature to see in this a genuine evolution if not of the law, at least of the judicial language, since other decisions refer not to bodies but to the 'dead' or to 'victims'. Thus, in its consideration of the facts in *Kamuhanda*, the ICTR Trial Chamber noted that 'Prosecution Witness GEA testified that he could not say how many people had died at that location, because "that day there were very many"'.[16]

Similarly, Pre-Trial Chamber II of the ICC has explained that 'for the act of murder to be committed the victim has to be dead and the death must result from the act of murder'.[17]

The human body and the fate inflicted on it are also absent from the definition of the crime of persecution, which, however, directly concerns the treatment of the body before death, the victimized individual being expelled from both the social and the living spheres. This characteristic has not gone unnoticed by judges and several decisions handed down by the ICTR and the ICTY explicitly define the purpose of the crime of persecution as being the removal of people from society:[18]

> When examining some of the examples of persecution mentioned above, one can discern a common element: those acts were all aimed at singling out and attacking certain individuals on discriminatory grounds, by depriving them of the political, social, or economic rights enjoyed by members of the wider society. The deprivation of these rights can be said to have as its aim the removal of those persons from the society in which they live alongside the perpetrators, or eventually even from humanity itself.[19]

Any explicit reference to the human body is likewise absent from the definitions of the crimes against humanity of enslavement and sexual slavery, whose essence nonetheless lies in considering the body as an object: as confirmed by the ICC's 'Elements of Crimes', enslavement and sexual slavery stem from the fact that '[t]he perpetrator exercised any or all of the powers attaching to the right of ownership over one or more persons, such as by purchasing, selling, lending or bartering such a person or persons, or by imposing on them a similar deprivation of liberty'.[20] This ownership and the 'objectification' of the body in the context of these crimes have been further explained in the case law and, in its *Kunarac* decision, the ICTY Appeals Chamber clearly specified that:

> the traditional concept of slavery, as defined in the 1926 Slavery Convention and often referred to as *'chattel* slavery', has evolved to encompass various contemporary forms of slavery which are also based on the exercise of any or all of the powers attaching to the right of ownership. In the case of these various contemporary forms of slavery, the victim is not subject to the exercise of the more extreme rights of ownership associated with 'chattel slavery', but in all cases, as a result of the exercise of any or all of the powers attaching to the right of ownership, there is some destruction of the juridical personality; the destruction is greater in the case of 'chattel slavery' but the difference is one of degree. The Appeals Chamber considers that, at the time relevant to the alleged crimes, these contemporary forms of slavery formed part of enslavement as a crime against humanity under customary international law.[21]

In this respect, it seems appropriate to note that the body as an object of which criminals dispose is a notion which remains implicit in the definition of the crime of enforced disappearance, for which the ICC's 'Elements of Crimes' document merely refers to the fact that '[t]he perpetrator [a]rrested, detained, or abducted one or more persons'.[22]

But where the law ceases to be implicit and treats the human body – and even the human anatomy – and its 'being taken possession of' as legal ingredients of the crime is in the definition of sexual violence. In relation to the crime against humanity of rape, the 'Elements of Crimes', probably inspired by the *Akayesu* precedent, repeatedly insists on the word 'body':

> The perpetrator *invaded the body* of a person by conduct resulting in penetration, however slight, of any part of the body of the victim or of the perpetrator with a sexual organ, or of the anal or genital opening of the victim with any object or any other part of the body.[23]

In the *Katanga and Ngudjolo Chui* case, the ICC Pre-Trial Chamber upheld this definition of rape[24] and, applying it to the facts of the case, reached the conclusion that:

there is sufficient evidence to establish substantial grounds to believe that members of the FNI and FRPI, by force or threat, *invaded the body, or parts of it, of women and girls abducted* before, during and after the February 2003 attack on the village of Bogoro.[25]

It is here interesting that the Chamber noted the significance not only of the body of the victims but also that of the criminals:

> The Chamber also finds that there is sufficient evidence to establish substantial grounds to believe that these rapes resulted in the *invasion of the body* of these civilian women by the penetration *of the perpetrator's sexual organ or other body parts*.[26]

The 'invasion of the body' by other bodies' parts as constituting the crime against humanity of rape is also found in the *Bemba Gombo* case, where the Pre-Trial Chamber of the ICC found that:

> Having reviewed the Disclosed Evidence ..., the Chamber finds that they consistently describe the multiple acts of rape they directly suffered from and detail *the invasion of their body by the sexual organ of MLC soldiers*, resulting in vaginal or anal penetration. The evidence shows that direct witnesses were raped by several MLC perpetrators in turn, that their clothes were ripped off by force, that they were pushed to the ground, immobilised by MLC soldiers standing on or holding them, raped at gunpoint, in public or in front of or near their family members.[27]

Judges also distinguish sexual violence perpetrated on living bodies from that perpetrated on dead ones, thereby affording protection not only to the human being but also to human dignity:

> the Chamber found that on 28 June 1994, near the Technical Training College, the Accused ordered Interahamwe to undress the body of a Tutsi woman, whom he called 'Inyenzi', who had just been shot dead, to fetch and sharpen a piece of wood, which he then instructed them to insert into her genitalia. This act was then carried out by the Interahamwe, in accordance with his instructions.
>
> The Chamber finds that the acts committed with respect to Kabanda and the sexual violence to the dead woman's body are acts of seriousness comparable to other acts enumerated in the Article, and would cause mental suffering to civilians, in particular, Tutsi civilians, and constitute a *serious attack on the human dignity* of the Tutsi community as a whole.[28]

This express reference to human dignity as a value to protect is a judicial innovation, the notion of human dignity being only implicit in the prohibition and punishment of crimes of mass violence. The

ICTR Trial Chamber thus proceeds here to a somewhat extended reading of the legal text insofar as it explicitly considers a 'serious attack on human dignity' as an inhumane act, although this appears nowhere in the definition of the crime. Indeed, considering the charge of inhumane acts as a crime against humanity, the Chamber found that:

> In respect of this count, the Accused must be found to have participated in the commission of inhumane acts on individuals, being acts of similar gravity to the other acts enumerated in the Article, such as would cause serious physical or mental suffering or constitute a serious attack on human dignity.[29]

This concern for the protection of human dignity is repeatedly found in decisions related to sexual violence, in the context of which, as mentioned above, the human body predominantly features. Could there be a legal link between the human body and human dignity? Could the human body be judicially considered as the guardian and receptacle of human dignity – the value to protect? This extract from the *Kajelijeli* decision handed down by Trial Chamber II of the ICTR would tend to go in that direction:

> The Chamber finds that these acts constitute a *serious attack on the human dignity of the Tutsi community as a whole*. Cutting a woman's breast off and licking it, and piercing a woman's sexual organs with a spear are nefarious acts of a comparable gravity to the other acts listed as crimes against humanity, which would clearly cause great mental suffering to any members of the Tutsi community who observed them. Furthermore, given the circumstances under which these acts were committed, the Chamber finds that they were committed in the course of a widespread attack upon the Tutsi civilian population.[30]

Could the human body thus be the shield of human dignity, the last protective bulwark of the value to protect? When the human body is targeted, martyred, destroyed, does it not become the irrefutable, tangible proof of the attack made on human dignity – or literally of the crime against humanity?

The body as evidence

If the idea developed here concerns mass violence in the sense of crimes against humanity and genocide, the probative value of the treatment and destruction of the victims' bodies is perhaps better revealed in the case of genocide. The definition of the crime of genocide, as enshrined in article 2 of the 1948 Genocide Convention – and reproduced verbatim in the Statutes of the International Criminal Tribunals and of the ICC – covers a whole range of genocidal acts that nonetheless remain unspecified. If it seems clear that these acts refer to the physical integrity of the person, the human body as such is not explicitly mentioned therein. In law, the crime of genocide –

> means any of the following acts committed with intent to destroy, in whole or in part, a national, ethnical, racial or religious group, as such:
> (a) Killing members of the group;
> (b) Causing serious bodily or mental harm to members of the group;
> (c) Deliberately inflicting on the group conditions of life calculated to bring about its physical destruction in whole or in part;
> (d) Imposing measures intended to prevent births within the group;
> (e) Forcibly transferring children of the group to another group.[31]

With respect to genocide, the ICC's 'Elements of Crimes' also refers to the physical integrity of the person – an expression that is to be found in the enumeration of prohibited acts under the category of 'causing serious bodily harm to members of the group', for which it is specified that '[t]he perpetrator caused serious bodily ... harm to one or more persons'.[32] Referring slightly more explicitly to human anatomy, the case law had already established that 'to a large extent, "causing serious bodily harm" is self-explanatory. This phrase could be construed to mean harm that seriously injures the health, causes *disfigurement* or causes any serious injury to the *external, internal organs or senses*.'[33] In a similar vein, the concept of physical destruction features expressly in the definition of the crime of 'deliberately inflicting on the group conditions of life calculated to bring about its physical destruction in whole or in part'.[34]

If physical destruction is thus explicitly present in the definition of the crime of genocide, this is not the case for the human body. If it is true that physical destruction encompasses an assault on the human body, the absence from the definition of the word 'body' and of any reference to its treatment by the *génocidaires* remains an unfortunate lacuna, precisely because the body is at the core of the criminal enterprise. The *génocidaire* fantasizes a body with various particularities on the basis of which the group targeted for annihilation is defined and differentiated. The bodies are marked with distinctive signs. Need one recall the ignoble yellow star? The bodies and the faces of the individuals are mocked, caricatured, mistreated, dehumanized and then destroyed. This has a very precise objective: to remove all traces of the existence of the group targeted for destruction, including in the bodies of the individuals, including in their human aspects.

The Nazi *univers concentrationnaire*, to adopt the expression of David Rousset,[35] planned precisely to orchestrate this dehumanization via fury directed against the body of the victims arrested and deported. 'The greatest enterprise of dehumanization of all times'[36] operated through atrocious brutalities inflicted on the bodies of the victims. They found themselves dispossessed of every personal effect, including their clothes, that is to say the social covering of the body; their hair was shaved; and their names were replaced by numbers, sometimes branded directly on the skin. The bodies of the victims were stripped of all human physical aspects before they were robbed of all living physical aspects, as is well captured by Ariane Kalfa:

> What is new and specific to concentration camps is the transformation of human beings into living cadavers. The frontier between life and death having ceased to be identifiable, man loses all dignity.... The anonymity of death in Auschwitz, the impossibility of distinguishing whether a prisoner was alive or dead, all this is worse than death and pushes the prisoner into the 'sub-humanity' to which Nazism destined him.[37]

The extreme violence of genocidal death culminates in the total destruction of the physical appearance of the victims and their bodies. It is more than a pathological outburst of violence. Rather, it is the destruction of the existence of the victims as human beings, the annihilation of their identity so as to wipe them out, including from both individual and collective memories. Destruction of the bodies is a purposeful act perfectly in tune with the genocidal modus operandi. Not only does it destroy life; it also destroys death. Once the life and death of the victims are annihilated, the existence of the targeted group is highly endangered, to the point of eradication. This idea has been perfectly expressed by Hélène Piralian:

> what genocide makes impossible and destroys is, we have to repeat it: Death itself, that is to say the possibility to symbolize death, the death of a has-been-alive who, after being part of the community of the living, would be part of that of the dead, thus making his death and mourning possible for his children who may then take over from him, as is the destiny of all humans.[38]

In an analysis of this 'killing of death' specific to the crime of genocide, Kalfa argues – very aptly – that destruction of death represents 'the physical annihilation of the existence of millions of individuals, and thus of the very idea of humanity itself':

> The industrial production of death where individuals are de-individualized, where subjectivity is annihilated, shows that death has become very different. Because what can the facts of transforming individuals into living skeletons and of reducing living human beings to ashes and smoke actually mean? What can the fact of erasing all traces, 'the memory and grief of the persons' who have loved those who have died signify? What is the sense of the censorship of the terms 'death' or 'victim' and of the imposition of the word 'Figuren' as a substitute, if it is not the sentencing to death of death, which is neither a metaphor nor a linguistic figure, but the physical annihilation of the existence of millions of individuals, and thus of the very idea of humanity itself?[39]

It is absolutely not by chance that, in all genocidal instances, the bodies of the victims are martyred to the point of becoming unknowable, that is to say unrecognizable. The destruction of their bodies denies the victims any belonging both to the targeted group and to the broader group of human beings. The *génocidaires* exclude their victims from the human sphere through the destruction of their physical appearance and bodily covering, thereby erasing every trace of the existence of their victims and facilitating their total eradication from individual and collective memories. Indeed, if the victims are physically destroyed, if their bodies become unrecognizable and unidentifiable as human corpses, thus impeding their incorporation into the human race, every trace of their passage on earth will disappear with their bodies. This disappearance puts into question the very existence of the group in the sense that, if there are no victims, there can no longer be an original group and furthermore no descendants. How could the group continue to exist in new generations if there never was a group? Piralian, in her study of the Armenian genocide, has explained that:

> The breaking up of the corpses into unnameable, that is to say unidentifiable, unattributable, pieces means that these pieces cannot be reunited in a nameable corpse of a 'has-been-alive' to whom a history could be given back. *This breaking up is pivotal for the perpetration of genocide as it concretely orchestrates the pulverization of the identities, excluding the targeted being from the human order as well as all possibility for him of any descendance. The crucial matter here is therefore, far beyond the incorporation of a loved one for whom mourning was made impossible (due to the misfortunes of his family's history), the pulverization and the destruction of the very link that unites a subject with his loved ones as, in the place of loved ones, there remains only an*

> *anonymous corpse, the same for all, made of all these disparate pieces which strew the deportation paths.* Under the weight of this violence, of this willingness to destroy, it is then the whole personal genealogical link of the individuals which finds itself broken and unreachable and the total link with the past is destroyed. In other words, *it is the scattering of unrecognizable corpses which makes impossible the constitution of identification links.*[40]

Further, by denying the existence of the victims through the destruction of their physical human aspects, the perpetrators leave the door open for the continued perpetration of the crime, through its denial. By denying the crime, deniers deny that there ever were victims and thereby question the existence of the victim group as such. According to their sordid reasoning, the absence of human bodies implies the absence of crimes and they will either minimize the real number of victims or bring about the conclusion that genocide was in fact never committed, paradoxically allowing it to continue. Both the reduction of the number of victims – which denies the reality of some victims and thus of some crimes – as well as the blatant and flagrant denial of the whole genocide proceed with the same intent: to ensure the ongoing annihilation of the group. According to Piralian:

> As a matter of fact, this disappearance of the dead, which consists in pretending that no living human being is dead but that, as having never existed, cannot be dead, casts new light on the burning controversy surrounding the number of deaths caused by a genocide as, in this case, to reduce the number of deaths means reducing the number of living who had existed, sustaining their disappearance and not registering their death. The reduction of the number of deaths should therefore not be understood as the parameter of a disaster but as an indirect means of continuing the disappearance of as many individuals as possible from the have-been-alive so that they also disappear from memories. Because how could we remember individuals who have never existed and how, in turn, could one deprived of antecedents exist? Where would he come from? ... In that sense, the denial of the number of deaths is part of the genocidal project as this backwards interpretation of time is nothing but an attempt to erase the origins.[41]

The goal of the destruction of the body is thus twofold: not only does it enable the criminals to erase all traces of their crimes; it also allows them to pursue their destructive and genocidal behaviour. Beyond the evident and barbarous violence of the acts perpetrated, the destruction of the human bodies responds to a clearly defined objective: the destruction of the group as such. In other words, the destroyed body matches both the genocidal modus operandi and the genocidal intent. It also provides irrefutable proof of the crime. From a practical perspective, this is not without consequence, since it raises the problems of how to reconcile the absence of the body, since it is destroyed, with the rules of evidence; and how to prove the existence of something that no longer exists.

If the letter of the law neglects to expressly consider the human body and its destruction as proofs of the crime perpetrated, the International Criminal Tribunals did, however, not hesitate to consider that the absence of the bodies or their non-identification was no barrier to the characterization of the crime. For instance, to prove that murder had been committed as a crime against humanity, the ICC insisted on the fact that:

> In determining whether the legal requirements of the act of murder as a crime against humanity are met, the Chamber points out the Prosecutor's obligation to provide the particulars in the charging document when seeking to prove that the perpetrator killed specific individuals. While the Chamber concedes that *there is no need to find and/or identify the corpse*, the Prosecutor is still expected to specify, to the extent possible, *inter alia*, the location of the alleged murder, its approximate date, the means by which the act was committed with enough precision, the circumstances of the incident and the perpetrator's link to the crime.
>
> However, the Chamber bears in mind the evidentiary threshold to be met at the pre-trial stage – 'substantial grounds' threshold – and the fact that *in case of mass crimes, it may be impractical to insist on a high degree of specificity*. In this respect, it is not necessary for the Prosecutor to demonstrate, for each individual killing, the identity of the victim and the direct perpetrator. Nor is it necessary that the precise number of victims be known. This allows the Chamber to consider evidence referring to 'many' killings or 'hundreds' of killings without indicating a specific number.[42]

It is true that this is a decision relative to murder as a crime against humanity and not to genocide, but the finding of the Court that 'in case of mass crimes, it may be impractical to insist on a high degree of specificity' is valid in both categories of crimes. Further, decisions of the ICTY concerning Srebrenica and those of the ICTR concerning Rwanda's genocide understand the treatment of the human body as proof of the crime. They rely especially on the existence and use of the means of destruction implemented by the criminals, thereby defeating the 'impracticalities' generated by evidentiary rules.

If the judgments on the crime of genocide handed down by the ICTR are numerous, the *Akayesu* case, as the first decision of the kind on the international scene, is of particular import. While it provided the Tribunal with an opportunity to define and interpret the applicable law, it is of the utmost interest in the context of the present analysis that the Trial Chamber gave a predominant place to the treatment of the human body as an integral part of the criminal modus operandi. This clearly stems from the testimonies heard by the Chamber in which the words 'bodies' and 'corpses' – used interchangeably – recur on many occasions. Dr Zachariah, then a member of Médecins Sans Frontières, notably reported the fate inflicted on the victims' bodies:

> He described in great detail the *heaps of bodies* which he saw everywhere, on the roads, on the footpaths and in rivers and, particularly, the manner in which all these people had been killed. At the church in Butare, at the Gahidi mission, he saw many wounded persons in the hospital who, according to him, were all Tutsi and who, apparently, had sustained wounds inflicted with machetes to the face, the neck, and also to the ankle, at the Achilles' tendon, to prevent them from fleeing.[43]

He likewise testified on the piles of bodies crowded along the roadsides:

> All the way through we could see on the ... hillside, where there were communities, people ... being pulled out by people with machetes, and we could see piles of bodies. In fact the entire landscape was becoming spotted with *corpses*, with *bodies*, all the way from there until almost Burundi's border.[44]

Dr Alison Desforges told of the Tutsi victims' bodies thrown into the river to 'send the Tutsi back to their place of origin'.[45] Cameraman and photographer Simon Cox filmed the practice,[46] while journalist Lindsey Hilsum testified on what she saw at the morgue: '*a big pile like a mountain of bodies* outside and these were bodies with slash wounds, with heads smashed in, many of them naked, men and women'.[47]

These testimonies, far from remaining dead letter, have been used by the Trial Chamber to prove the genocidal intent to destroy the Tutsis. In particular, the wounds to the Achilles' tendon observed by Zachariah did not go unnoticed by the Chamber, which inferred from them 'the resolve of the perpetrators of these massacres not to spare any Tutsi. Their plan called for doing whatever was possible

The human body: victim, witness and evidence 69

to prevent any Tutsi from escaping and, thus, to destroy the whole group.'[48]

Despite the fact that the qualification of genocide is a rarer occurrence at the ICTY, this does not mean it is non-existent. In its first finding of genocide, in the *Krstić* case, the ICTY Trial Chamber made a clear reference to the human body and its treatment by expressly recording the scientific analysis of the evidentiary elements related to the executions carried out in Srebrenica:

> The extensive forensic evidence presented by the Prosecution strongly corroborates important aspects of the testimony of survivors from the various execution sites. Commencing in 1996, the Office of the Prosecutor (hereafter 'OTP') conducted exhumations of 21 gravesites associated with the take-over of Srebrenica.... Of the 21 gravesites exhumed, 14 were primary gravesites, where bodies had been put directly after the individuals were killed. Of these, eight were subsequently disturbed and bodies were removed and reburied elsewhere, often in secondary gravesites located in more remote regions. Seven of the exhumed gravesites were secondary burial sites.[49]

In order to prove the crime of genocide, the Chamber then reported in detail the medico-legal analyses, thereby linking the treatment of the human body to the crime perpetrated. The Chamber was thus able to establish that the great majority of the victims were male; this was a decisive element in this case for the qualification of genocide, the men of Srebrenica having been targeted to ensure the extinction of the group as a whole:

> The forensic evidence supports the Prosecution's claim that, following the take-over of Srebrenica, thousands of Bosnian Muslim men were summarily executed and consigned to mass graves. Although forensic experts were not able to conclude with certainty how many bodies were in the mass graves, due to the level of decomposition that had occurred and the fact that many bodies were mutilated in the process of being moved from primary to secondary graves by mechanical equipment, the experts were able to conservatively estimate that a minimum of 2,028 separate bodies were exhumed from the mass graves.
>
> ...
>
> The forensic examinations of the gravesites associated with Srebrenica reveal that only one of the 1,843 bodies for which sex could be determined was female. Similarly, there is a correlation between the age distribution of persons listed as missing and the bodies exhumed from the Srebrenica graves: 26.4 percent of persons listed as missing were between 13–24 years and 17.5 percent of bodies exhumed fell within this age group; 73.6 percent of persons listed as missing were

over 25 years of age and 82.8 percent of bodies exhumed fell within this age group.[50]

The Chamber was thus able to observe that:

> Overall the Trial Chamber finds that the forensic evidence presented by the Prosecution provides corroboration of survivor testimony that, following the take-over of Srebrenica in July 1995, thousands of Bosnian Muslim men from Srebrenica were killed in careful and methodical mass executions.[51]

The Chamber turned to the medico-legal analysis carried out on the cadavers to determine the sex of the victims but also to be able to classify the victims as civilian members of a group destined for destruction – another requirement of the crime of genocide:

> The results of the forensic investigations suggest that the majority of bodies exhumed were not killed in combat; they were killed in mass executions. Investigators discovered at least 448 blindfolds on or with the bodies uncovered during the exhumations at ten separate sites. At least 423 ligatures were located during exhumations at 13 separate sites. Some of the ligatures were made of cloth and string, but predominately they were made of wire. These ligatures and blindfolds are inconsistent with combat casualties. The Prosecution also relied on forensic evidence that the overwhelming majority of victims located in the graves, for whom a cause of death could be determined, were killed by gunshot wounds. The exhumations also revealed that some of the victims were severely handicapped and, for that reason, unlikely to have been combatants.[52]

The Chamber, here demonstrating a particular interest in the treatment of cadavers and especially their concealment, further confirmed the non-combatant character of the victims:

> Most significantly, the forensic evidence presented by the Prosecution also demonstrates that, during a period of several weeks in September and early October 1995, Bosnian Serb forces dug up many of the primary mass gravesites and reburied the bodies in still more remote locations.... The reburial evidence demonstrates a concerted campaign to conceal the bodies of the men in these primary gravesites, which was undoubtedly prompted by increasing international scrutiny of the events following the take-over of Srebrenica. Such extreme measures would not have been necessary had the majority of the bodies in these primary graves been combat victims.[53]

The significance of the treatment of the human body in the establishment of evidence in the context of genocide was later reiterated in the judgment when the Chamber explicitly linked the fate inflicted on the victims' bodies with the crime perpetrated:

> One hundred and fifty bodies were recovered from the mass grave and the cause of death for 149 was determined to be gunshot wounds. All were male, with a mean age from 14 to 50 and 147 were wearing civilian clothes. Forty-eight wire ligatures were recovered from the grave, about half of which were still in place binding the victims' hands behind their backs. Experts were able to positively identify nine of the exhumed bodies as persons listed as missing following the take-over of Srebrenica. All were Bosnian Muslim men.[54]

It is noteworthy in this respect that the Chamber devoted an entire part of its decision to the reburials,[55] with the consideration that:

> The forensic evidence presented to the Trial Chamber suggests that, commencing in the early autumn of 1995, the Bosnian Serbs engaged in a concerted effort to conceal the mass killings by relocating the primary graves to remote secondary gravesites.[56]

Thanks to its consideration of the human bodies of the victims, the Trial Chamber 'concluded that almost all of those murdered at the execution sites were adult Bosnian Muslim men and that up to 7000–8000 men were executed'[57] and that '[a] crime of extermination was committed at Srebrenica'.[58] Most interestingly, it also inferred genocidal intent from the treatment of the bodies:

> Finally, there is a strong indication of the intent to destroy the group as such in the concealment of the bodies in mass graves, which were later dug up, the bodies mutilated and reburied in other mass graves located in even more remote areas, thereby preventing any decent burial in accord with religious and ethnic customs and causing terrible distress to the mourning survivors, many of whom have been unable to come to a closure until the death of their men is finally verified.[59]

The International Criminal Tribunals have thus been able to take into account the destruction of and treatment inflicted on the victims' bodies not only to characterize the massacre as such, but also to qualify it legally. The subsequent identification of the bodies conducted thanks to medico-legal analyses made it possible to establish whether those victims belonged to a civilian population targeted for crimes against humanity or to a group destined for genocide. More fundamentally, the judicial consideration and scientific analysis of the bodies brought the victims back into the sphere of the 'have-been-alive',[60] and endowed them with a humanity they had in reality never lost.

Conclusion

Robert Antelme wrote in his moving testimony:

> All of us are here to die. That's the objective the SS have chosen for us. They haven't shot us, they haven't hanged us; but, systematically deprived of food, each of us, whether it be sooner or later, must become the dead man they have aimed at. So each of us has as his sole aim to prevent himself from dying. The bread we eat is good because we are hungry. But while it assuages hunger, we also know, we also sense that with bread life maintains itself in our bodies. The cold is painful, but the SS want us to die from the cold, and we have to protect ourselves from it, because death is what's in the cold. Work is exhausting and – for us, it is absurd – but its effect is to wear, and the SS want us to die from work, and so it is that when we work we must be sparing of ourselves, because death is what's in the work. And then there's time. The SS believe we'll end up dying from not eating, or from working; the SS believe they'll get us through weariness – that is, through time. Death is what's in time.[61]

'Life maintains itself in our bodies' … the perpetrators of mass violence, crimes against humanity, and genocides, know it, so much so that it is this full awareness of this life, of this humanity of their victims which drives them to destroy their bodies. Mass violence and the 'destructiveness of bodies' (*destructivité des corps*), to adopt the expression of Jacques Sémelin,[62] are intrinsically bound. As this chapter has attempted to demonstrate, the destruction of the human body is the proof of the perpetration of mass violence; it is also its essential corollary, since it is this destruction that renders mass violence possible. Sémelin has perfectly identified the 'destructiveness of bodies' as 'the means by which the perpetrators create for themselves a radical *psychic distance* from their victims, to convince themselves that they are not, that they are no longer human beings'.[63] He explains that:

> The practice of massacre confirms *a contrario* one of the strongest affirmations of the philosopher Emmanuel Levinas, namely that recognition of our shared humanity necessarily comes through the face to face encounter. Even if the enemy is depicted by propaganda under hideous and threatening traits, he retains a terribly human face. Hence, this is why the perpetrator of the massacre must as speedily as possible 'disfigure' this other likeness to fend off any risk of identification. To be able to kill him implies dehumanizing him, no more 'solely' by the make-believe of the propaganda, but now through acts: cut his nose or ears, for immediate reassurance that he no longer has a human face.

The cruelty is truly a mental operation on the body of the other aimed at smashing his humanity....
This spiral of destructiveness of the bodies may be pursued even after death. The bodies, even deprived of life, may still resemble those of the living. So they must be scalped, shrivelled, crushed so that they no longer resemble anything.[64]

If it is true that the international criminal norm has a lacuna in this respect, if it is true that the very concept of 'human body' is only subsidiary in the definitions of the crimes and if it is equally true that the treatment of the victims' bodies by the criminals is not subject to specific legal provisions, it is also true that international criminal justice has no less integrated 'body' into its language and has explicitly regarded the fate inflicted on the victims' bodies as a means of proving crimes against humanity and genocides. If the impact of the terminology used by the International Criminal Tribunals and by the ICC remains difficult to evaluate and if their use of the word 'body' may simply respond to a purely narrative purpose of window-dressing, the value of the contribution of the case law on the treatment of the human body is more easily measurable. It clearly corresponds to a judicial effort aimed, if not at making the law evolve, at least at better grasping the very essence of mass violence, and perhaps at attempting to comprehend the incomprehensible.

Notes

1 The text of this chapter was translated from the author's French by Cadenza Academic Translations.
2 That is not to say that the crimes are systematically deprived of all economic, patrimonial or cultural dimensions. For instance, the crime of persecution 'may manifestly encompass various forms and does not require a physical element'. ICTY, *Prosecutor v. Kupreškić* (case no. IT-95-16), Judgment, Chamber II, 14 January 2000, para. 568. For confirmation, see ICTY, *Prosecutor v. Vasiljević* (case no. IT-98-32-T), Judgment, Chamber II, 29 November 2002, para. 246, and ICTR, *Prosecutor v. Semanza* (case no. ICTR-97-20-T), Judgment and sentence, Chamber III, 15 May 2003, para. 348. The crime of 'persecution' encompasses not only bodily and mental harm and infringements upon individual freedom but also acts that appear less serious, such as those targeting property, so long as the victimized persons were specially selected on grounds linked to their belonging to a particular community. ICTY, *Prosecutor v. Blaškić* (case no. IT-95-14-T), Judgment, Chamber I, 3 March 2000, para. 233. Yet, the individual human being

primarily benefits from legal protection. The judicial processes conducted by the Allied Powers Under Control Council Law No. 10 in Germany clearly show that the human being – and not property – was regarded as the potential victim of the acts recognized as crimes against humanity. See notably *United States v. Flick et al.* (the '*Flick* case'), case no. 5, Military Tribunal IV, 1947, in *Trials of War Criminals Before the Nuremberg Military Tribunals Under Control Council Law No. 10* (Washington, US Department of the Army, Government Printing Office, 1946–49), vol. 6, p. 1215. This aspect became even more evident with the definition of the crime of genocide, which exclusively protects the individual as a member of the group and excludes any economic, patrimonial or cultural consideration. Targeting groups is the characteristic of this crime, as the *travaux préparatoires* of the Convention on the Prevention and Punishment of the Crime of Genocide and the debates on the possible inclusion of cultural genocide therein clearly indicate. Polish lawyer Raphaël Lemkin, who coined the term 'genocide', had identified 'genocide in the cultural field' as 'the prohibition or the destruction of cultural institutions and cultural activities, of the substitution of education in the liberal arts for vocational education, in order to prevent humanistic thinking, which the occupant considers dangerous because it promotes national thinking'. R. Lemkin, *Axis Rule in Occupied Europe: Laws of Occupation, Analysis of Government, Proposals for Redress* (Washington, DC: Carnegie Endowment for International Peace, Division of International Law, 1944), pp. xi–xii. The initial text of the Genocide Convention – that of the human rights division of the Secretariat – included cultural genocide among the acts of genocide and defined it as the destruction of the specific characteristics of the groups persecuted via various methods, such as enforced exile, prohibition of the use of national language, destruction of books and similar acts. Draft Convention, UN Doc. A/AC.10/41 and UN Doc. A/362 (appendix II). The subsequent text of the ad hoc Committee had addressed the issue of cultural genocide in its article III. Nevertheless, in addition to its arguable lack of definitional clarity, this clause was far from gaining unanimous support. The majority of representatives felt that including cultural genocide would weaken the Convention, whose aim was to prevent and punish mass murder. As the ICTY trial observed in the *Krstić* case, 'Although the Convention does not specifically speak to the point, the preparatory work points out that the "cultural" destruction of a group was expressly rejected after having been seriously contemplated'. *Prosecutor v. Krstić* (case no. IT-98-33), Judgment, Chamber I, 2 August 2001, para. 576. See also *Prosecutor v. Brđanin* (case no. IT-99-36-T), Judgment, Chamber II, 1 September 2004, para. 694. The Genocide Convention excludes cultural genocide from its ambit to maintain the focus on the protection of the individual and the only reference to this form of genocide is found in the criminalization of the enforced transfer of children, which effectively constitutes a direct threat to the cultural survival of the group.

The human body: victim, witness and evidence   75

3 Article 7 of the Rome Statute of the ICC, 17 July 1998, UN Doc. A/CONF.183/9.
4 Article 6 of the Rome Statute.
5 It may be noted that judgments make interchangeable use of the words 'body' and 'corpse', even if it is generally understood that 'corpse' refers to a dead body.
6 Translation by the author. The original version reads: 'In der Todesdrohung, die ich zum erstenmal in voller Deutlichkeit beim Lesen der Nürnbergergesetze verspürte, lag auch das, was man gemeinhin die methodische 'Entwürdigung' der Juden durch die Nazis nennt. Anders formuliert: der Würdeentzug drückte die Morddrohung aus.' J. Améry, *Jenseits von Schuld und Sühne: Bewältigungsversuche eines Überwältigten* (Munich: Szczesny, 1966), p. 137.
7 Article 7 of the Rome Statute.
8 Article 7 of the Rome Statute also prohibits 'severe deprivation of *physical* liberty'. Emphasis added.
9 Report of the Preparatory Commission for the International Criminal Court, Part II: Finalized draft text of the 'Elements of Crimes', 2 November 2000, PCNICC/2000/1/Add.2, in *Official Records of the Assembly of States Parties to the Rome Statute of the International Criminal Court, First Session, New York, 3–10 September 2002* (United Nations publication, sales no. E.03.V.2 and corrigendum), part II.B (henceforth 'Elements of Crimes'), article 7-1-k. Emphasis added.
10 Ibid., Article 7-1-f-1.
11 Ibid., Article 7-1-g-4-1.
12 Ibid., Article 7-1-g-5-1. Emphasis added.
13 Ibid., Article 7-1-a.
14 Ibid., Article 7-1-b.
15 ICTR, *Prosecutor v. Akayesu* (case no. ICTR-96-4-T), Judgment, Trial Chamber I, 2 September 1998, paras 201–10, 277, 280, 288, 290, 297, 304, 307, 322.
16 ICTR, *Prosecutor v. Kamuhanda* (case no. ICTR-99-54A-T), Judgment and sentence, Trial Chamber II, 22 January 2004, para. 345. Emphasis added.
17 ICC, *Prosecutor v. Bemba Gombo* (case no. ICC-01/05-01/08), Decision pursuant to article 61(7)(a) and (b) of the Rome Statute on the charges of the prosecutor against Jean-Pierre Bemba Gombo, Pre-Trial Chamber II, 15 June 2009, para. 132. Emphasis added.
18 Ibid.
19 Ibid.
20 'Elements of Crimes', articles 7-1-c-1 and 7-1-g-2-1.
21 ICTY, *Prosecutor v. Kunarac et al.* (case nos IT-96-23 and IT-96-23/1-A), Judgment, Appeals Chamber, 12 June 2002, para. 117. Emphasis added.
22 'Elements of Crimes', article 7-1- i-1-a.
23 Ibid., article 7-1-g-1-1. Emphasis added. See also ICTR, *Prosecutor v. Akayesu*, note 15, paras 596–7 and 686–8; ICTY, *Prosecutor v. Furundžija* (case no. IT-95-17/1), Judgment, Trial Chamber II, 10 December 1998, paras 174, 176 and 181.

24 ICC, *Prosecutor v. Katanga and Ngudjolo Chui* (case no. ICC-01/04-01/07), Decision on the confirmation of charges, Pre-Trial Chamber I, 30 September 2008, para. 438. Emphasis added.
25 Ibid., para. 442. Emphasis added. Both the FNI (Front des Nationalistes et Intégrationnistes; Front of Nationalists and Integrationists) and the FRPI (Force de Résistance Patriotique en Ituri; Ituri Patriotic Resistance Force) refer to armed militias.
26 Ibid., para. 351. Emphasis added.
27 ICC, *Prosecutor v. Bemba Gombo*, note 31, para. 165. Emphasis added. The MLC (Mouvement de Libération du Congo; Movement for the Liberation of Congo) is a political party in Democratic Republic of the Congo presided by Jean-Pierre Bemba Gombo.
28 ICTR, *Prosecutor v. Niyitegeka* (case no. ICTR-96-14-T), Judgment and sentence, Trial Chamber I, 16 May 2003, paras 463 and 465. Emphasis added.
29 Ibid., para. 460.
30 ICTR, *Prosecutor v. Kajelijeli* (case no. ICTR-98-44A-T), Judgment and sentence, Trial Chamber II, 1 December 2003, para. 936. Emphasis added.
31 Article 6 of the Rome Statute.
32 'Elements of Crimes', article 6-b-1.
33 ICTR, *Prosecutor v. Kayishema and Ruzindana* (case no. ICTR-95-1-T), Judgment, Trial Chamber II, 21 May 1999, para. 109. Emphasis added. For confirmation, see ICTY, *Prosecutor v. Krstić*, note 2, para. 510.
34 See 'Elements of Crimes', article 6-c-4. See also ICTR, *Prosecutor v. Akayesu*, note 15, paras 505–6; ICTR, *Prosecutor v. Kayishema and Ruzindana,* note 35, para. 116.
35 D. Rousset, *L'Univers concentrationnaire* (Paris: Les Editions de Minuit, 1965).
36 A. Frossard, *Le Crime contre l'humanité* (Paris: Editions Robert Laffont, 1987), p. 42.
37 A. Kalfa, *La Force du Refus: philosopher après Auschwitz* (Paris: L'Harmattan, 2004), pp. 138–9. Translation by the author. The original version reads: 'Ce qui est nouveau et spécifique aux camps de concentration est le fait que des êtres humains soient transformés en cadavres-vivants. La frontière entre la vie et la mort n'étant plus identifiable, l'homme perd toute dignité.... L'anonymat de la mort à Auschwitz, l'impossibilité de distinguer si un prisonnier était mort ou vivant, tout cela est pire que la mort, et fait basculer le prisonnier dans la "sous-humanité" à laquelle le nazisme le destinait.'
38 H. Piralian, *Génocide et transmission* (Paris: Editions L'Harmattan, 1994), pp. 33–4. Translation by the author. The original version reads: 'ce que le génocide rend impossible et détruit c'est, répétons-le: la Mort même, c'est-à-dire la possibilité de symbolisation de la mort, celle d'un ayant-été-vivant qui, après avoir fait partie de la communauté des vivants, ferait partie de celle des morts permettant que, pour ses enfants, sa mort et son deuil soient possibles et qu'ainsi ils puissent lui succéder, comme c'est le destin de tout humain'.

39 Kalfa, *La Force du Refus*, note 39, pp. 139–40. Footnote omitted. Translation by the author. The original version reads: 'La production industrielle de la mort où les individus sont désindividualisés, la subjectivité anéantie, montre que la mort est devenue tout autre. Car, que peut signifier le fait de transformer des individus en cadavres vivants, et des êtres humains vivants en cendre et en fumée? Que peut signifier le fait d'effacer toutes les traces, "le souvenir et le chagrin des personnes" qui ont aimé ceux qui sont morts? Quel est le sens de la censure du terme de "mort" ou de "victime", et du fait d'imposer celui de "Figuren" comme substitut, si ce n'est la mise à mort de la mort, ce qui n'est pas une métaphore, ni une figure de style, mais l'anéantissement physique de l'existence de millions de personnes et par la même de l'idée d'humanité.'

40 Piralian, *Génocide et transmission*, note 40, p. 33. Translation by the author. The original version reads: 'Le morcellement des corps en morceaux innommables, c'est-à-dire non identifiables, non attribuables fait que ces morceaux ne peuvent être réunis en un corps nommable d'un "ayant-été-vivant" à qui pourrait être rendue une histoire. *Ce morcellement est un des pivots du génocide en ce qu'il est mise en place concrète de la pulvérisation des identités, excluant celui qui en est l'objet de l'ordre de l'humain comme de toute possibilité pour lui de descendance.* Ce dont il s'agit est donc, bien au-delà de l'incorporation d'un être cher dont le deuil aurait été rendu (à cause des avatars de son histoire familiale) impossible pour un sujet, la pulvérisation et la destruction du lien même qui unit un sujet à ses êtres aimés puisqu'en place des êtres chers de chacun ne reste plus qu'un corps anonyme, le même pour tous, fait de ces morceaux disparates qui jonchent les chemins de déportation. Sous le poids de cette violence, de cette volonté de destruction, c'est alors tout le lien généalogique personnel des sujets qui se trouve brisé et hors d'atteinte et le lien total au passé emporté. Autrement dit, *c'est l'éparpillement des corps rendus ainsi méconnaissables qui rend impossible la constitution des liens identificatoires.*' Original emphasis.

41 Ibid., p. 52. Translation by the author. The original version reads: 'cette disparition des morts qui consiste à faire en sorte qu'il n'y ait pas mort de vivants mais que ceux-ci n'ayant jamais existé ne puissent être morts, éclaire d'un jour nouveau la brûlante polémique autour du nombre des morts d'un génocide, puisqu'en ce cas, réduire le nombre des morts, c'est réduire le nombre des vivants ayant existé, soutenir leur disparition et non inscrire leur mort. La réduction du nombre des morts ne serait plus alors à entendre comme le paramètre d'un désastre plus ou moins grand mais bien comme une manière détournée de continuer à faire disparaître le plus de personnes possibles des ayant-été-vivants pour qu'elles disparaissent également des mémoires. Car comment pourrait-on se souvenir de personnes n'ayant jamais existé et comment celui qui n'a pas d'antécédent pourrait-il exister à son tour? D'où viendrait-il? … En ce sens, le déni du nombre des morts fait bien partie du projet génocidaire, puisqu'en prenant ainsi le temps à rebours, c'est bien d'une tentative d'effacement des origines mêmes dont il s'agit.'

42 ICC, *Prosecutor v. Bemba Gombo*, note 18, paras 133–4. Footnotes omitted. Emphasis added.
43 ICTR, *Prosecutor v. Akayesu*, note 15, para. 115. Emphasis added.
44 Ibid., para. 158. Emphasis added.
45 Ibid., para. 120. Emphasis added.
46 Ibid., para. 161.
47 Ibid., para. 160.
48 Ibid., para. 119. See also J. Sémelin, *Purify and Destroy: The Political Uses of Massacre and Genocide* (trans. C. Schoch) (New York: Columbia University Press, 2007), p. 357.
49 ICTY, *Prosecutor v. Krstić*, note 2, para. 71.
50 Ibid., paras 73–4.
51 Ibid., para. 79.
52 Ibid., para. 75.
53 Ibid., para. 78.
54 Ibid., para. 202. See also paras 208–24, 222–3, 229–30, 237–8, 250.
55 Ibid., paras 257–61.
56 Ibid., para. 257.
57 Ibid., para. 487.
58 Ibid., para. 505.
59 Ibid., para. 596.
60 Piralian, *Génocide et transmission*, note 40, p. 33.
61 R. Antelme, *The Human Race* (trans. J. Haight & A. Mahler) (Evanston: Marlboro Press/Northwestern, 1992), pp. 39–40.
62 Sémelin, *Purify and Destroy*, note 50, p. 352.
63 Ibid. Original emphasis.
64 Ibid., pp. 351–2.

Bibliography

Améry, J., *Jenseits von Schuld und Sühne: Bewältigungsversuche eines Überwältigten* (Munich: Szczesny, 1966)
Antelme, R., *The Human Race* (trans. J. Haight & A. Mahler) (Evanston: Marlboro Press/Northwestern, 1992)
Frossard, A., *Le Crime contre l'humanité* (Paris: Editions Robert Laffont, 1987)
Kalfa, A., *La Force du Refus: philosopher après Auschwitz* (Paris: L'Harmattan, 2004)
Lemkin, R., *Axis Rule in Occupied Europe: Laws of Occupation, Analysis of Government, Proposals for Redress* (Washington, DC: Carnegie Endowment for International Peace, Division of International Law, 1944)
Piralian, H., *Génocide et transmission* (Paris: Editions L'Harmattan, 1994)
Rousset, D., *L'Univers concentrationnaire* (Paris: Les Editions de Minuit, 1965)
Sémelin, J., *Purify and Destroy: The Political Uses of Massacre and Genocide* (trans. C. Schoch) (New York: Columbia University Press, 2007)

The human body: victim, witness and evidence 79

International legislation

Convention for the Prevention and Punishment of the Crime of Genocide, United Nations, 1948. Approved and proposed for signature, ratification or accession by the General Assembly of the United Nations, Resolution 260 A (III) of 9 December 1948 (entry into force 12 January 1951)

Draft Convention on the Crime of Genocide, General Secretariat of the United Nations, 26 June 1947, UN Doc. A/AC.10/41

Draft Convention on the Crime of Genocide, United Nations General Assembly, Note by the Secretary General, 25 August 1947, UN Doc. A/362 (appendix II)

Report of the Preparatory Commission for the International Criminal Court, Part II: Finalized draft text of the 'Elements of Crimes', 2 November 2000, PCNICC/2000/1/Add.2, in *Official Records of the Assembly of States Parties to the Rome Statute of the International Criminal Court, First Session, New York, 3–10 September 2002* (United Nations publication, sales no. E.03.V.2 and corrigendum), part II.B ('Elements of Crimes')

Rome Statute of the International Criminal Court, Adopted by the United Nations Diplomatic Conference of Plenipotentiaries on the Establishment of an International Criminal Court on 17 July 1998, UN Doc. A/Conf.183/9, 1998

Statute of the International Tribunal for the former Yugoslavia, United Nations, 1993. Approved by the Security Council of the United Nations in Resolution 827 of 25 May 1993

Statute of the International Tribunal for Rwanda, United Nations, 1994. Decided by the Security Council of the United Nations, Resolution 955 of 8 November 1994

ICC (International Criminal Court)

Prosecutor v. Bemba Gombo (case no. ICC-01/05-01/08), Decision pursuant to article 61(7)(a) and (b) of the Rome Statute on the charges of the prosecutor against Jean-Pierre Bemba Gombo, Pre-Trial Chamber II, 15 June 2009

Prosecutor v. Katanga and Ngudjolo Chui (case no. ICC-01/04-01/07), Decision on the confirmation of charges, Pre-Trial Chamber I, 30 September 2008

ICTR (International Criminal Tribunal for Rwanda)

Prosecutor v. Akayesu (case no. ICTR-96-4-T), Judgment, Trial Chamber I, 2 September 1998

Prosecutor v. Kajelijeli (case no. ICTR-98-44A-T), Judgement and sentence, Trial Chamber II, 1 December 2003

Prosecutor v. Kamuhanda (case no. ICTR-99-54A-T), Judgment and sentence, Trial Chamber II, 22 January 2004

Prosecutor v. Kayishema and Ruzindana (case no. ICTR-95-1-T), Judgment, Trial Chamber II, 21 May 1999

Prosecutor v. Niyitegeka (case no. ICTR-96-14-T), Judgment and sentence, Trial Chamber I, 16 May 2003

Prosecutor v. Rutaganda (case no. ICTR-96-3-T), Judgment, Trial Chamber I, 6 December 1999

Prosecutor v. Semanza (case no. ICTR-97-20-T), Judgment and sentence, Trial Chamber III, 15 May 2003

ICTY (International Criminal Tribunal for the former Yugoslavia)

Prosecutor v. Blaškić (case no. IT-95-14-T), Judgment, Trial Chamber I, 3 March 2000

Prosecutor v. Brđanin (case no. IT-99-36-T), Judgment, Trial Chamber II, 1 September 2004

Prosecutor v. Delalić et al. (case no. IT-96-21), Judgment, Trial Chamber, 16 November 1998

Prosecutor v. Furundžija (case no. IT-95-17/1), Judgment, Trial Chamber II, 10 December 1998

Prosecutor v. Krstić (case no. IT-98-33), Judgment, Trial Chamber I, 2 August 2001

Prosecutor v. Kunarac et al. (case nos IT-96-23 and IT-96-23/1-A), Judgment, Appeals Chamber, 12 June 2002

Prosecutor v. Kupreškić (case no. IT-95-16), Judgment, Trial Chamber II, 14 January 2000

Prosecutor v. Vasiljević (case no. IT-98-32-T), Judgment, Trial Chamber II, 29 November 2002

Nuremberg Military Tribunals Under Control Council Law No. 10

United States v. Flick et al. The '*Flick* case', case no. 5, Military Tribunal IV, 1947, in *Trials of War Criminals Before the Nuremberg Military Tribunals Under Control Council Law No. 10* (Washington: US Department of the Army, Government Printing Office, 1946–49), vol. 6, p. 1215

4

Moral discourse and action in relation to the corpse: integrative concepts for a criminology of mass violence

Jon Shute

Introduction: the moral–emotional 'work' of serious crime in peacetime and in conflict

In stable, late-modern societies, crimes are adjudicated breaches of morality formally defined in law. They are variable in content across place and time, and do not always have a readily identifiable victim or definitions that have the informal moral support of the population; however, many of the most serious offences against the person and property commonly evoke moral outrage in onlookers and deliver emotional trauma to victims.[1] Their commission requires at least one perpetrator to be not bound by the moral–emotional content of the law at the time of the offence, nor by the likely consequences of their actions on the emotional life of others. The perpetrator will nonetheless spend most time conforming to most laws and, moreover, is statistically more likely to witness and experience the types of trauma associated with the victim;[2] this points both to the dangers of essentializing and othering 'the criminal', and also to the complexities of the moral–emotional 'work' carried out in the service of crime. Regardless of one's immediate status in the perpetrator–victim–onlooker nexus, immoral (criminal) action must be emotionally neutralized and/or cognitively reframed as contextually acceptable, and the emotional trauma of its consequences managed in order to minimize psychological harm.

Serious crime is definitive of contexts of mass violence, where the rule of law collapses and agents of state control are often prime perpetrators. In such contexts, organized mass perpetration creates distinct classes of the gravest offences[3] and both bystanding and victimization are commensurately endemic. In any given theatre of conflict, there is, therefore, an unquantifiable amount of individual and collective moral transgression and associated emotional trauma to negotiate and manage. While it is possible that non-lethal violence is more common than lethal violence in such contexts, the latter and its prime 'product' – the corpse – create specific and ongoing sets of moral–emotional problems that demand further analysis. Not only must one explain the crimes inherent in the production of the corpse (that is, homicide), but one must also account for the morally difficult task of corpse disposal by perpetrators, onlookers and the families of victims. Furthermore, in an age when advances in forensic techniques render sites of disposal and the corpse itself increasingly 'eloquent', the post-conflict investigation of atrocity may reactivate trauma and force actors implicated in murder to revisit and modify narratives of moral denial. In contexts where some form of transitional justice is possible, corpses may be used in the service of re-moralizing post-conflict society, whether evidentially in forensic settings, or symbolically in commemorative rituals and sites. In societies that experience no or inadequate transitional justice, the absence or attentional neglect of the corpse may act as a focal point for continued and contested moral discourse, often many years after the original conflict.

This brief sketch has been intended to make two points: first, that all serious crime entails significant moral–emotional 'work', both in the foreground of the offence and in its diffuse emotional aftermath; and second, that the material human remains of lethal mass violence possess the capacity to greatly extend that 'work' in ways that have a significance well beyond the original crime(s). This chapter develops these ideas to argue that the moral discourse and action surrounding the production and treatment of corpses is, in a general sense, beneficial for an understanding of the long-term trajectory of societies affected by mass violence; and in a more specific sense, beneficial to the formulation of a nascent criminology of atrocity and transitional justice. Beginning with a contextualizing survey of the puzzlingly 'light' engagement of criminology – the study of crime – with the crimes of mass violence, the chapter describes important themes in what might be called 'moral arousal management theory': that body of interdisciplinary theory that attempts to understand the ways in which the moral–emotional 'work' of crime is performed and managed. When applied to the production and treatment of corpses, the conceptually integrative potential of the theory – across moral actors, time and levels of analysis – is then elaborated, and key research questions derived. Before the conclusion, the chapter discusses the core methodological and ethical issues involved in establishing a criminology of the corpse and mass violence, and its place in the wider process of re-ascribing value to radically devalued human lives.

Criminology's historical engagement with the corpse and mass violence

Engaging the corpse

The corpse *qua* corpse has never been a central object of criminological study and, as such, there is no 'criminology of the corpse'. This is not to say that human remains have not featured in 140 years of criminological enquiry, as two temporally polar examples illustrate. First, in the late nineteenth century, the criminal anthropology of Cesare Lombroso[4] and his *scuola positiva* was foundational to criminology and made intensive use of the body parts of dead criminals. The epiphanic moment that inspired Lombroso's biosocial theory of criminality came from his inspection of the skull of a 'brigand', and skeletons gathered from private collections formed both the raw data for measurement and analysis, and the pedagogical tools that aided disciplinary development. Lombroso's methods and theories quickly became discredited; however, *in vivo* anthropometry continued and survives today in 'bio-criminological' research.[5] Second, the dying and dead body of the criminal has also featured in late-modern analyses of historical trends in western punishment. For example, several authors[6] have followed sociologist Norbert Elias in his account of the 'civilizing process' and noted how changing sensibilities born of broader sociocultural developments have made once-common public corporal and capital violence (including corpse defilement) unacceptable.[7]

In these examples, however, it will be seen that the corpse is not central to the intellectual project but a means to a more distant explanatory end – a useful but peripheral object from which inferences can be drawn about criminals or society. Moreover, there is no substantive criminological literature on the corpse of the *victim*;

analyses of patterns in the post-mortem treatment of homicide victims tend to be performed by forensic scientists or psychologists. This lack of substantive interest in the corpse as an object of enquiry most likely results from the central disciplinary focus on the *criminal* and the homicidal *act*, as opposed to the *product* of the act, which, in keeping with this legalistic focus, tends to be seen mainly for its evidentiary value.

Engaging mass violence

The criminological literature in relation to mass violence can be organized crudely into three broad periods. The first runs roughly from the publication of the first edition of Lombroso's *L'Uomo deliquente* in 1876 until 1942. This period is characterized by the *absence* of discourse on mass violence, with virtually all the energies of the developing discipline focused on establishing the principles and methods of biological, psychological and sociological variants of criminological positivism. While there is little to no *explicit* reference to mass violence, biological criminology, based as it was in assumptions of inherited and acquired pathology, species regression and a within-race hierarchy of physical–moral types, articulated well with the dominant racist–eugenicist colonial mind-set that violently repressed and exploited so-called 'lesser' peoples. Its methods were also taken up avidly in Weimar Germany and later National Socialist Germany,[8] where elastic terms such as 'asocial' and 'criminal type', along with the pseudo-science of racial assessment and categorization, were placed firmly in the service of peacetime terror and wartime genocide. As some late-modern criminologists have noted, criminology during this period was often *complicit* in the discourse and practices of mass violence.[9]

The second broad period of criminological literature runs from 1943 to 1989 and began with the publication of a series of works by Sheldon Glueck that emerged from his role as a US delegate involved in the planning of the Nuremburg Military Tribunal.[10] This marked the first substantive – even seminal – practical engagement of a criminologist with mass violence, though it is notable that Glueck's activity was both short-lived and set apart from his main career interests, which were in delinquent development. He is now better known, ironically, for work on somatotyping[11] (criminal body shape), which was very much in a Lombrosian tradition that maintained peripheral credibility only in the USA after the Second World War. The Holocaust also motivated a small number of other articles in criminology journals in the late 1940s,[12] as did the Eichmann trial in the early 1960s,[13] but it is very clear that, unlike in history, political science and social psychology, there was an effective non-engagement of academic criminology with the subject matter. In its post-war obsession with juvenile delinquency, it is as if the discipline as a whole turned its back on the mass crimes of the previous generation, to focus on the relatively petty crimes of the next. A small number of works[14] in the 1970s and 1980s applied radical (often Marxist) and rights-based critiques to the traditional concerns, methods and definitions of a perceived 'establishment' criminology, and attempted to switch the focus to crimes of power and of the powerful. This occasionally involved discussion of mass violence but it was seldom, if ever, its sole object.

The final, productive period of criminological literature runs roughly from 1990 to the present day and is characterized by a greater disciplinary reflexivity and, led by a number of notable scholars, a progressive engagement in the substance of mass violence. While the critical criminologists of the 1970s and 1980s paved the way for greater disciplinary self-awareness, a number of publications at the turn of the century dealt explicitly with criminology's non-engagement with mass violence.[15] Two principal sets of factors can be identified. First, criminology, by being driven to a great extent by criminal justice policy and practice, has been accused of being too concerned historically with the 'internal' matters of the nation-state and/or its constituent federal jurisdictions. It has, then, been both inward-looking and neglectful of crime with an international dimension or in other (particularly non-western) jurisdictions, and too accepting of establishment definitions of crime. It has, in other words, been too long interested in the state-defined crimes of the powerless as opposed to the state-led crimes of the powerful; and again, one encounters accusations of disciplinary conservatism and complicity. A second, related reason for non-engagement is the suspicion that criminology may be poorly equipped to study crimes of mass violence and, in that sense, have 'little to offer'. Mass violence is argued by some to be too great in scale, too complex, too dynamic and too dangerous to study using habitual survey and interview methods, and too conceptually alien, with its notions of collective, ideologically driven intent and state-legitimized violence.

If these perceived disciplinary limitations help to explain historical non-engagement, two further factors are required to explain more recent and sustained *engagement*. The first concerns sets of changes and developments that have been *internal* to the discipline. As criminology has expanded, diversified and become more intellectually mature, there has perhaps been a greater willingness – and institutional space – to challenge its foundational concerns and shibboleths. The US debate over the nature of and duty to realize a 'public sociology' has also spilled over into criminological discourse[16] and – in England and Wales as elsewhere – major funding sources with smaller budgets and universities competing in an increasingly commercialized environment have all tended to demand greater public engagement and demonstration of concrete research 'impact'. At the same time, improved communications and funding for collaboration have created and sustained a range of international networks and professional societies. Together, these trends have motivated criminologists to look beyond their traditional territorial as well as thematic boundaries, and rewarded them for novel, collaborative and progressive international research.

All of these changes have not, of course, *automatically* resulted in research interest in mass violence, and a second set of factors *external* to the discipline have arguably provided the real impetus for criminological engagement. As Hagan has noted, the context of the Cold War perhaps promoted a degree of isolationism in western criminology, which began to break down with the dismantling of state communism.[17] This new order provided opportunities to study violence associated with the collapsed regimes but was also associated with the return of major international crimes to the European mainland, in Bosnia and Kosovo, and coincided with both the genocide in Rwanda and the deeply contested 'war on terror'. At the same time, international responses to these and other contexts of mass violence, such as the International Criminal Tribunals on both the former Yugoslavia (ICTY) and Rwanda (ICTR), the Truth and Reconciliation Commission in post-apartheid South Africa, and associated major developments in international law, have occurred.

In short, the last twenty-five years have witnessed a more confident, critical, connected and outward-looking criminology, engaging with the sometimes disturbingly plentiful 'raw materials' of mass crime and international justice associated with profound historical events and transitions. While far from 'mainstream', there are now substantive works associated with conceptual variants of mass violence: state crime;[18] international and supranational crime;[19] and atrocity crimes and transitional justice.[20] Examples of dedicated institutions,[21] journals,[22] book series[23] and international networks[24] can all now be described.

Engaging corpses of mass violence

As might be expected from the foregoing discussion, the criminological intersection of the Venn diagram of 'corpses' and 'mass violence' is small indeed, and while a stimulating recent period of the work of the penologist David Garland[25] deals with the dead and dying body in two large-scale 'institutions' of American violence – public torture lynching and capital punishment – the focus is again not on the corpse *qua* corpse, nor on phenomena that might be universally recognized as mass violence. Only Wayne Morrison's work on historical representations of the corpse within and without criminology inhabits this liminal intellectual space.[26]

In summary, this section has shown that while it is no longer possible to bemoan the complete neglect by criminology of mass violence in its various forms, it must also be acknowledged that this engagement has been very recent indeed, and is so far from the disciplinary 'mainstream' that it is still associated with a relatively small network of named academics. There is, therefore, only a nascent 'criminology of mass violence', with much debate over the precise nature and scope of the subject matter, as well as over its organizing frameworks, priorities and methods of study. To understand why this has been the case, and why there has been until now no attendant work on the millions of corpses resulting from mass violence, requires a return in great measure to our main interest: the moral–emotional 'work' of serious crime and its consequences. As we shall see in the next section, some of the most important criminological work emerging in recent years has attempted to understand the 'management' of this work, but it is equally clear that, to the extent that the discipline has been complicit in or has wilfully ignored historical mass violence, it has arguably employed similar sets of 'denial' strategies that have rendered it, at best, an academic bystander or, at worst, a 'fellow traveller' or even active collaborator in mass violence.

Moral transgression and moral arousal management: a master concept?

Despite the phenomenal scale and complexity of the task, a prime question arising out of every context of mass lethal violence is 'how could this happen?' Scholars with a wide variety of intellectual and methodological traditions have focused their explanatory lens on one or more of the conventional triad of moral actors (perpetrators, bystanders, victims), on different levels of analysis (macro-, meso-, micro-) and on the particularity or generality of the subject matter. There is, therefore, a rich canon of theory beyond the scope of this chapter including: climate change; 'hard times'; historic group enmities; modernist objectivity; bureaucratic rationality; militarist authoritarianism; eliminationist ideology; obedience to authority; group conformity pressures, etc. This section seeks to cut across these diverse literatures to focus on the moral–emotional work carried out in the commission and aftermath of the serious crimes of mass violence. *Crimes of mass violence* are taken here to include the organized crimes of international law defined in the Rome Statute[27] – genocide, crimes against humanity, war crimes and the crime of aggression – in addition to the myriad individual criminal acts necessitated by them and occurring as a consequence of intra- and inter-state conflict. It is assumed here that all such offences occasion serious moral transgression, and, even if sanctioned situationally at the time, are taught to be *generally* morally reprehensible in the peacetime moral education and moral discourse of most societies. Serious moral transgression of this order is conceived to occasion strong emotions that must be overcome (or harnessed) to commit the act, or to witness the act without taking preventive action, and that are felt by all actors, including the living victim, both at the time of the offence and in its aftermath. These emotions vary in strength and nature (terror, dread, excitement, helplessness, fury) across moral actors and may best be grouped under a more neutral, technical term: *moral arousal*, that is, the physiological arousal that is cognitively interpreted as subjective emotion in moral contexts. It is to be expected that moral arousal varies significantly across persons, situations, contexts and over time (for example, through repeat exposure) but is never conceived to be trivial. This section, then, reframes the 'moral work' of the crimes of mass violence as *moral arousal management*, a term that is also used to organize a range of cognate theories with disparate roots and applications. What follows is a brief review of key ideas in this literature, leading to a discussion of their application to mass violence.[28]

Psychoanalytic approaches: denial

Modern work on the management of troubling realities begins, of course, with Sigmund Freud and his intellectual as well as literal descendants. The term 'denial' and phrase 'to be in denial' have escaped psychotherapy to become understood in the vernacular as an unwillingness to engage – cognitively, emotionally or behaviourally – with something one knows one should. As is typical for 'escaped' technical vocabulary, the original meaning is debased, and the 'something' one should act on is often relatively trivial (recent weight gain, a work deadline, a painful tooth). While Freud has been noted[29] to write inconsistently over his career on the subject, denial (*Verleugnung*, also translated as 'disavowal') is generally taken to be one of several psychic defence mechanisms by which the ego protects itself against emotionally harmful external realities. It can be distinguished from repression, which is a set of defences against the instinctual demands of the id, but, like repression, is conceived to be a fundamentally unconscious process. Some of Freud's most extensive but arcane writing on the subject is in the realm of psychosexual development ('penis envy' and so forth[30]), and while the details need not detain us here, the process and products of denial, like repression, could become pathological for the individual, resulting in mental distress in later life and requiring insight therapy. The concept has *not* been applied extensively within psychotherapy to crime or crimes of mass violence and is noted here primarily for its foundational historical value: it makes clear that there are external realities that can be emotionally overwhelming and that must be managed psychologically in order to avoid or minimize harm. The fact that Freud was not himself always clear on the meaning of the term and that it is difficult, if not impossible, to empirically test or refute should not detract either from its value as metaphor, or from its subsequent influence.

Socio-criminological approaches: moral neutralization

As Copes and Maruna note,[31] psychoanalytic notions seem to have been unacknowledged influences on what might be termed the first and foremost work in the sociology/criminology of denial: Gresham Sykes and David Matza's classic 1957 paper outlining the 'techniques of neutralization' employed by urban delinquents in the service of criminal conduct.[32] At a time when leading subcultural theories of delinquency posited anti-establishment, pro-criminal sets of values and beliefs, the authors were interested in explaining why their research interviews indicated that most delinquents displayed pervasively conventional attitudes and behaviour most of the time.

Sykes and Matza posited that, instead of understanding morals as absolutes, delinquents rationalized their behaviour *situationally*, such that the moral problems of offending were 'neutralized' in specific settings in predictable ways: denial of responsibility; denial of injury; denial of victim; condemning the condemners; appeal to higher loyalties. The techniques are perpetrator-focused and are conceived to be both preparatory and subsequent to the offence; that is, they 'free up' the otherwise conventional young person to offend, and are systematized as rationalizations after the offence. The ability of suggestible and fatalistic working-class youths to tread the line between deviance and conformity Matza later described as 'drift'.[33]

A full conceptual–empirical review is beyond the scope of this chapter; however, there is modest to good support for the theory across a range of studies examining a range of offences, and it has also been extended by Agnew to victimization as a set of internal coping dimensions.[34] For our purposes, however, it is important to note the techniques as means by which moral arousal, albeit for relatively petty offences in heavily contextualized settings, can be managed and minimized.

Social cognitive approaches: moral disengagement and cognitive transformation

Social psychology offers a wide range of theories that can be seen to be relevant to the management of moral arousal, so much so that we are here able to give only an outline of selected concepts.

Albert Bandura's work on 'moral disengagement' may be seen to be a synthetic approach that combines the author's own sociocognitive theory with insights from a range of other social psychological concepts, and that arrives at some similar conclusions to Sykes and Matza.[35] The theory describes the internal mental processes by which individuals disengage from the self-censure associated with the commission of immoral ('inhumane') acts. Four broad sets of processes are described: reframing of immoral acts as morally worthy; disavowal of personal moral agency; minimizing the consequences of the act; and denigrating the victim. The commission of a range of criminal and immoral acts has been empirically demonstrated to be strongly associated with the tendency to disengage from the moral content of behaviour in these ways.[36]

One other, distinctively sociocognitive criminological contribution in recent years has been Shadd Maruna's work[37] on narrative accounts of criminal persistence (the long-term maintenance of a criminal lifestyle) and criminal desistence (the permanent cessation of offending). Maruna shifts focus from the synchronic employment of cognitive techniques that sidestep the moral problems of offending, to the diachronic employment of cognitive techniques that help make sense of a criminal past and distance it in such a way that the offender is able to 'make good' and extinguish a previous criminal identity. In an in-depth qualitative longitudinal study[38] of repeat adult offenders in Liverpool, England, Maruna found that men who persisted in a life of crime created and pursued 'condemnation scripts': systematized understandings of themselves and the world around them based in anger, futility and resignation. This was in contrast to men who did not deny their past behaviour but who creatively reinterpreted it as not being reflective of the core, 'real them', who was, and remained, capable of reform. These men – in Maruna's parlance, those following 'redemption scripts' – were much more likely to desist from offending. This draws attention to some of the temporal *dynamics* of moral reasoning and describes a paradox whereby strategies of cognitive distortion that have been used in the past to successfully manage the moral problems of offending may, in modified form, also be harnessed to achieve permanent desistance from offending.

One seemingly obvious limitation of this literature in relation to the concept of moral arousal management is that it is predominantly – some might say excessively – cognitive, and there is little overt reference to the emotional content of the immoral act. Cognition and emotion have long been seen to be intimately coupled, however, and although the former is afforded primacy, it is clear that the modes of thought described above have the effect of licensing feelings of righteousness and revenge, and minimizing or deflecting self-censure and its associated feelings of guilt, blame and personal failure. These are, to quote Bollas in Cohen, 'troubling emotional recognitions, of which one needs to be innocent'.[39]

Applications to mass violence

Thus far, the survey of moral arousal management in relation to crime has been restricted to relatively petty peacetime offending, but it is also a key theme in more recent accounts of mass violence.

Here, we discuss some important contributions of just two authors, in roughly chronological order. First, the magisterial work of the late sociological criminologist Stan Cohen must be recognized. In a series of articles culminating in the 2001 book *States of Denial*, Cohen, reflecting on his upbringing in apartheid South Africa and later residence in Israel at the time of the first Palestinian Intifada, analysed diverse 'denial' literatures and applied them to massive human rights abuses. He found such literatures important for understanding and confronting these abuses and made at least three distinctive contributions.[40]

First, the focus of the book is not primarily on the perpetrator, but on the *bystander* at various levels of analysis, including those proximate to and with demonstrable knowledge of an atrocity, but also more distal state-level observers in the international community. Cohen developed and extended Matza's concept of 'subterranean values' – the coincidence of the moral neutralization techniques of delinquents with the reasoning of juvenile justice actors and the content of substantive legal defences – to posit *cultures of denial*: routinized and immersive habits of moral non-engagement with the suffering of often distant (non-western) peoples and nations.

Second, Cohen refined the modes of bystander denial to three basic types and gave instances of transitions between them in contexts of mass violence: literal denial ('it could not have happened'); interpretative denial (euphemistic relabelling of acknowledged acts); and implicatory denial (minimization or indifference to the moral consequences of an acknowledged act).

Finally, Cohen focused on modes of *acknowledgement* designed to combat and reverse these denial strategies (for example, those employed by campaigning humanitarian agencies) and called for more systematic efforts at prevention via education, whistleblowing, and enforceable regulatory strategies. By drawing examples from numerous illustrative instances of verbal and written evidence from contexts of mass violence, Cohen convincingly extended the originally modest reach of much of the moral arousal management literature reviewed above.

The second author to make a distinctive sociocriminological contribution in this area is John Hagan. In a body of work spanning the mid to late 2000s, Hagan and colleagues employed innovative methods to the study of mass violence in Darfur, which employed elements of moral arousal management theory to substantiate allegations of state-led genocide.[41] Conceptually, the author specified a 'collective framing process' by which macro-level state propaganda consisting of Arab–Islamic supremacist and dehumanizing rhetoric conditioned and mobilized government-backed militia groups, and provided a vocabulary of motive that was employed in conflict with black African victims to commit and amplify genocidal violence. Methodologically, Hagan employed sophisticated multi-level statistics to analyse the results of a unique mixed-methods survey[42] of victimization in Chadian refugee camps – the Atrocities Documentation Survey of 1,136 survivors. Among a number of important findings, Hagan substantiated his macro–meso–micro conceptual model, and showed how the highest levels of recorded lethal and sexual violence occurred when government forces and militia attacked in tandem, and where a dehumanizing racial discourse ('We will kill all the men and rape all the women. We want to change the colour…') was most often heard. These findings helped to demonstrate, variously, both direct and indirect government involvement, an endemic ideological mass denial of victimhood, and the racialized both mens rea and actus reus of crime. The latter point is theoretically important as it demonstrates that moral neutralization/denial/arousal management is *preparatory* to serious crime, in addition to being a post hoc rationalization of it.

In summary, this section has outlined a rich and multi-disciplinary set of theories that all tend towards the explanation of how the moral arousal attendant on the commission and witnessing of crimes of varying severity can be actively managed, minimized, evaded or cognitively reframed as righteous. Such techniques are contended to be causally important at the time of the offence, but also in retrospect, in the service of the management of self-identity and moral agency. By extending the source theory to contexts of mass violence, criminologists have begun to challenge the disciplinary neglect of mass violence and to extend its conceptual and empirical boundaries. Moral arousal management may now be taken as a sine qua non for the occurrence of mass violence.

Integrative potential of moral arousal management in relation to the corpse

This section returns to the main conceptual task outlined in the introduction, namely, the extension of a moral arousal management perspective to the study of human remains produced as a consequence of mass violence. It is argued that moral discourse in relation to the corpse has the potential to integrate several important dimensions of conflict and, in so doing, to provide a novel and holistic framework for understanding organized atrocity. Three possibilities for integration are identified: across moral actors, levels of analysis and time.

Integration across moral actors

In contrast to the traditional concern of explaining the perpetration of mass violence, it is argued that a focus on its corporeal product temporally extends the moral arousal of killing beyond the original act and distributes it among all affected moral actors. To be sure, the same suite of moral arousal management techniques used to produce the corpse can also be applied to its disposal by perpetrators; the self-protective dehumanizing language/denial of victimhood used in torture and murder has also been used to process human remains, for example the common description of victims of extermination camps in Nazi-occupied Poland as 'rags', 'pieces' and 'dolls'.[43] This euphemistic labelling, combined with the use of living victims as intermediaries (the *Sonderkommando*) charged with the actual business of touching, transporting and destroying bodies via cremation, is argued to help relieve the moral problem of corpse disposal for the perpetrator. Knowledge of the production and destruction of corpses is also an important source of moral arousal for onlookers – those who are direct witnesses, who live in close proximity to the violence or who are charged officially or prudentially – for example in the context of very rapid mass killing such as the Rwandan genocide – with the task of burying abandoned corpses. Onlookers who benefit in some sense from the killing, for example the local residents who appropriated the houses of murdered Jews in Lanzmann's *Shoah*,[44] are likely to manage/neutralize a different range of moral problems to those negotiating the trauma of burying members of their own community or primary group. Finally, while the dead cannot, of course, engage with their murdered selves, the presence or indeed *absence* of the corpse produces secondary victimization and trauma among family members that must be managed as grief and a sense of profound injustice. As campaigning organizations such as the Mothers and Grandmothers of the Plaza Mayo illustrate in the context of the Argentinian 'Dirty War', family members may harness their grief for progressive purposes and, in so doing, become a force for acknowledgement in wider society.

Integration across levels of analysis

Moral discourse in relation to the corpse can also be seen at all three principal levels of analysis. At the macro (societal) level, the human remains of victims of mass violence can have an important evidentiary and symbolic role in transitional justice arrangements and in the related construction of official commemorative narratives. Bodies, for example those buried and reburied in mass graves after the fall of Srebrenica, may be used positively to challenge the denial narratives of perpetrators; in that example, bound and blindfolded corpses were in fact enemy combatants returning fire, and so forth. Human remains have also been employed variably but widely in sites of memory in Rwanda and Cambodia, and, in a different sense, Argentina, where an official sculpture park in Buenos Aires[45] offers meditation on the theme of absence, and former clandestine detention centres such as the Navy School of Mechanics (Escuela Superior de Mecánica de la Armada, or ESMA) have been converted to the headquarters of humanitarian and investigative agencies.

Moral arousal management in relation to the corpse can also be an important consideration at the meso (group, institutional) level. Staying with the Argentinian example, it is notable that the methods of corpse disposal outlined in *Nunca más*, the 1984 report from the National Commission on the Disappearance of Persons (Comisión Nacional sobre la Desaparición de Personas, or CONADEP),[46] seem closely related to the institutional habits and practices of the perpetrators. For example, staged shootings can be seen as extensions of the corrupt police practices of faking evidence, and the 'death flights' a relatively routine extension of the Navy's normal habits of transporting cargo over water. While such practices no doubt also reflect simple opportunity, it is possible that the reliance on peacetime operational routines and habits makes the moral problem of corpse handling and disposal cognitively and emotionally easier.

Finally, as detailed above, the micro level of analysis is also fundamental to understanding how individual moral actors participate – or decline to participate – in the process of corpse destruction and disposal.

Integration across time

One limitation of moral arousal management theories, with the exception of Maruna's aforementioned work on identity and criminal desistance, is that they tend to be synchronic and situational in focus, while, of course, mass violence necessitates complex multi-level process that have a historical context, a pathological present and a future legacy. Moral arousal management in relation to the corpse can speak to this temporal component in two ways.

First, the theories and principles described above can be applied to the structural and cultural *background*, the situational *foreground* and the varied *consequences* of mass violence. Thus, knowledge of the cultural and religious background of a given society can help us understand the value ascribed to the corpse in peacetime, together with the normal but variable practices of corpse handling and disposal; this, in turn, helps us to understand the extent to which these are employed or violated in times of conflict. We have discussed at length the primary importance of moral arousal management for handling the acute emotional demands of the production and disposal of the corpse in the phenomenological foreground of mass violence, and also indicated how that legacy can be extended and challenged by moral discourse in its aftermath.

The second relevant temporal aspect is perhaps more compelling, however, and relates to the different phases of the trajectory of the corpse itself: from *destruction*, through *identification*, to *commemoration* of the victims. If the production and destruction of the corpse can be seen as a radical devaluation of human life requiring moral arousal management, the search and identification phase represents an important counter-movement, and the beginning of the process of re-ascribing value. Agencies such as the International Commission on Missing Persons (ICMP[47]) in Sarajevo and the Argentine Forensic Anthropology Team (Equipo Argentino de Antropología Forense, or EAAF[48]) employ technologically sophisticated methods to locate, excavate and identify the human contents of mass graves. While the handling of these remains surely itself involves moral arousal management techniques, for example the development of technical objectivity and 'detachment', the work of such agencies is key, both to the evidentiary confrontation of perpetrator denial, and to the process of grieving for family members. Finally, the commemoration phase of the corpse's journey, for example via burial, collective ritual or monuments, can be seen to be approaching the full re-ascription of value to the deceased; however, the extent to which the psychotherapeutic analogue of 'closure' is experienced by families, communities and society as a whole is perhaps questionable. While a conventional view of commemoration might favour full acknowledgement of the past (an 'insight' model), examples of Holocaust survivors remaining silent about their experiences, or the controversies attendant on re-opening uninvestigated mass graves in Spain eight decades on from the killing, suggest that the further deployment of moral arousal management (a 'denial' model) may be considered preferable by those wishing to 'move on' from the violence.[49]

In summary, this section has described something of the integrative potential of moral discourse in relation to the human remains of mass violence. While necessarily speculative given the novelty of the subject matter, a range of empirical questions suggest themselves, and it is to the methodology required to explore these questions that we now turn.

Methodological and ethical issues in the study of moral arousal management and the corpse

Methodology

Criminology has been described as a 'rendezvous' discipline in that it had, until the recent advent of dedicated undergraduate degree programmes, been traditionally practised by academics with training in a related 'home' discipline such as sociology, law or psychology, and who imported the range of theories, perspectives and methods of that training to research common criminological concerns. As such, the phrase 'criminological research methods' tends to be something of a misnomer and, in practice, researchers use an eclectic range of quantitative, qualitative and mixed methods drawn from across the social sciences and humanities. Naturally, methods do not exist in the abstract but only in relation to concrete research questions. For the purposes of this section, then, it is proposed that a broad, two-part question suggests itself from the foregoing discussion: (1) Which accounts of moral arousal management best fit the treatment of corpses in a given context of mass violence, that is, across moral actors, levels of analysis and over time, and (2) to what extent are these accounts generalizable across contexts?

From first principles, two broad sets of empirical strategies suggest themselves, each, inevitably, with attendant limitations magnified by the very considerable general difficulties of researching mass violence.

The first and most obvious strategy is *retrospective* in nature and can be applied to any past or, perhaps more accurately, currently inactive theatre of violence. To the extent that moral arousal management is encoded and communicated in language, there are several forms of qualitative data that can be collected and analysed using standard deductive and inductive techniques. These include written texts in the form of archived bureaucratic documents (policies, orders, committee minutes, email threads, etc.), but also the proceedings and transcripts of trials and other arenas of transitional justice, for example the Argentinian *Nunca más*, or South African Truth and Reconciliation process.[50] Where documents and archives are very extensive, careful consideration of sampling procedures is needed in order to render the exercise both manageable and valid. Another option is to proactively collect retrospective interview data from a range of actors affected by lethal violence. One option here may be to attempt semi-structured or narrative professional interviews with actors involved in the investigation or commemoration processes, or to locate surviving family members involved in campaigning organizations. In theory, perpetrators may also be approached if they have been identified and are locatable, but here the central limitations of researching moral arousal management assert themselves: the painful nature of recollection, together with any tacitly agreed 'pact of silence', are likely to entail great difficulties in gaining access and, even if this could be arranged, tact and sensitivity would be required to elicit high-quality data.

If interviews do indeed prove difficult, the range and quality of secondary perpetrator datasets can sometimes be surprising, as Neitzel and Welzer's recent analysis of thousands of surveillance transcripts from Nazi prisoners of war has demonstrated;[51] these are *in vivo* conversations, often among fellow combatants, stripped of a layer of artifice and defence associated with interrogation.

Once datasets have been obtained, standard approaches[52] to analysis can be performed, including content analysis, which systematically derives codes from the definitive aspects of a given theory (for example the techniques of neutralization, or predicted elements of a condemnation script) and seeks confirmatory and disconfirmatory evidence across cases. A more inductive, grounded approach could, conversely, be used in order to evolve explanatory accounts of moral arousal management in relation to the corpse directly from the data.

Once a method is established, it would be of great interest to compare discourse relating to the same event from the perspective of different moral actors, at different levels of analysis (individual, near group, state) and for the same moral actors over time. A further step would be to take the findings from one context and see if they apply in another (part 2 of our over-arching research question).

The second fundamental research strategy is *prospective*, that is, to collect longitudinal data as some part of the process of recovery from mass violence proceeds. The most suitable methodological approach for this is ethnographic, where immersion can promote a deeper understanding of the context under study and help establish the networks of trust and rapport that facilitate the collection of valid observational and interview data. Work-shadowing of forensic science professionals is an example of the kinds of activity that could be undertaken. Short of full ethnography, attending a transitional justice arena as an observer in the manner of Hagan's work[53] on the functioning of the ICTY could also be beneficial. Similar options with regard to qualitative analysis of observational field notes are available.

Ethical issues

Most university research ethics committees and those of the principal national and international funding councils require a robust ethical engagement with standard issues when research examines human beings. These include: informed consent, considerations of researcher and participant safety, anonymity, data confidentiality and data security. These issues are rarely insurmountable; however, careful consideration would need to be given when researching the human remains of mass violence, given the emotional weight of the subject matter and the moral arousal experienced by the researcher and by the participant(s) reliving trauma. Careful thought would also need to be given to the safety of both researcher and participant, depending on the nature of the context and its proximity to active violence.

Conclusion

This chapter has made the case that after a long history of complicity and indifference, criminology has at last begun to see beyond its traditionally narrow concerns and engage substantively with mass violence. It has argued that contexts of mass violence are saturated with the heavy moral–emotional 'work' associated with overcoming the peacetime taboos attendant on committing serious crime, 'work' that must also be performed by the unresponsive bystander, and is experienced most directly as trauma by the victim at the time of the offence and in its aftermath. We have made the point that lethal violence produces a corpse and that the dynamic fate of this material fact has the potential to greatly extend the moral–emotional work of serious crime well beyond the original act.

After reviewing the suite of cognate theories that were deemed to assist in the management of moral arousal, we argued that their application to the corpse in contexts of mass violence had the potential to act as an integrative motif across moral actors, levels of analysis and over time. The moral–emotional work of a society coming to terms with a legacy of mass violence may be done, in other words, through the corpse. Finally, we offered some tentative suggestions for the textual analysis of documents and speech likely to contain evidence of moral arousal management, and posited both retrospective and prospective strategies for the ethical, competitive and comparative refinement of theory. There are profound but exciting challenges involved in taking this research agenda forward.

Notes

1 For an empirical confirmation across a range of countries, see J. van Kesteren, J. van Dijk & P. Mayhew, 'The international crime victim surveys', *International Review of Victimology*, 20 (2014), pp. 49–69.
2 See W. G. Jenning, A. R. Piquero & J. M. Reingle, 'On the overlap between victimization and offending: a review of the literature'. *Aggression and Violent Behavior*, 17 (2012), pp. 16–26.
3 Genocide, crimes against humanity.
4 C. Lombroso, *Criminal Man* (London: Duke University Press, 2006 – original edition 1876).
5 See N. Rafter, *The Criminal Brain: Understanding Biological Theories of Crime* (New York: New York University Press, 2008).
6 For example, P. Spierenburg, *Violence and Punishment: Civilising the Body* (Cambridge: Polity Press, 2013).
7 N. Elias, *The Civilising Process* (Oxford: Blackwell, 2000 – original edition 1939).
8 R. Wetzell, *Inventing the Criminal: A History of German Criminology 1880-1945* (Chapel Hill: University of North Carolina Press, 2000).
9 W. Morrison, *Criminology, Civilisation and the New World Order* (Abingdon: Routledge, 2006).

10 For example, S. Glueck, 'By what tribunal shall war offenders be tried?', *Harvard Law Review*, 56:7 (1943), pp. 1059–89; S. Glueck, *The Nuremburg Trial and Aggressive War* (New York: Knop, 1946).
11 E. Glueck & S. Glueck, *Physique and Delinquency* (New York: Harper, 1956).
12 For example, R. M. W. Kempner, 'Murder by government', *Journal of Criminal Law and Criminology*, 38:3 (1948), pp. 235–8; L. Alexander, 'Destructive and self-destructive trends in criminalised society: a study of totalitarianism', *Journal of Criminal Law and Criminology*, 39:5 (1949), pp. 553–64.
13 N. N. Kittrie, 'A post mortem of the Eichmann case – the lessons for international law', *Journal of Criminal Law and Criminology*, 55:2 (1964), pp. 16–28.
14 For example, T. Platt, 'Prospects for a radical criminology in the United States', *Crime and Social Justice*, 1 (1974), pp. 2–10.
15 For example, W. S. Laufer, 'The forgotten crime of genocide', in W. S. Laufer & A. Adler (eds), *Advances in Criminological Theory, Volume 8: The Criminology of Criminal Law* (New Brunswick: Transaction Publishers, 1999), pp. 71–82; L. E. Day & M. Vandiver, 'Criminology and genocide studies: notes on what might have been and what still could be', *Crime, Law and Social Change*, 34 (2000), pp. 43–59; G. S. Yacoubian, 'The (in)significance of genocidal behaviour to the discipline of criminology', *Crime, Law and Social Change*, 34 (2000), pp. 7–19.
16 I. Loader & R. Sparks, *Public Criminology?* (London: Routledge, 2011).
17 J. Hagan & W. Rymond-Richmond, *Darfur and the Crime of Genocide* (New York: Cambridge University Press, 2008).
18 P. Green & T. Ward, *State Crime: Government Violence and Corruption* (London: Pluto Press, 2004).
19 See A. Alvarez, *Governments, Citizens, and Genocide* (Bloomington: Indiana University Press, 2001); A. Smeulers & R. Haveman (eds), *Supranational Criminology: Towards a Criminology of International Crimes* (Oxford: Intersentia, 2008); J. J. Savelsberg, *Crime and Human Rights: Criminology of Genocide and Atrocities* (London: Sage, 2010).
20 S. Karstedt & S. Parmentier 'Introduction to the special issue', *European Journal of Criminology*, 9:5 (2012) (special issue, *Atrocity Crimes and Transitional Justice*), pp. 465–7.
21 See the International State Crime Initiative at http://statecrime.org/ (accessed 29 January 2014).
22 See http://statecrime.org/journal (accessed 29 January 2014).
23 See for example, Intersentia's series on transitional justice, at www.intersentia.co.uk/Serie.aspx?serieCode=STJ&langId=2 (accessed 29 January 2014).
24 See www.esc-eurocrim.org/workgroups.shtml#atrocity (accessed 29 January 2014).
25 D. Garland, *Peculiar Institution: America's Death Penalty in an Age of Abolition* (New York: Oxford University Press, 2010).
26 Morrison, *Criminology*.

27 The 1998 Rome Statute of the International Criminal Court, available at www.icc-cpi.int/nr/rdonlyres/ea9aeff7-5752-4f84-be940a655eb30e16/0/rome_statute_english.pdf (accessed 29 January 2014).
28 This review draws on S. Cohen, *States of Denial: Knowing About Atrocities and Suffering* (Cambridge: Polity Press, 2001); and S. Copes & S. Maruna, 'Excuses, excuses: what have we learned from five decades of neutralisation research?', in M. Tonry (ed.), *Crime and Justice: A Review of Research* (Chicago: University of Chicago Press, 2005), vol. 32, pp. 221–320.
29 See Cohen, *States of Denial*, p. 25.
30 S. Freud, 'Some psychical consequences of the anatomical distinction between the sexes', in *Standard Edition* (London: Hogarth Press, 1925), vol. 19, pp. 248–58.
31 Copes & Maruna, 'Excuses, excuses'.
32 G. M. Sykes & D. Matza, 'Techniques of neutralization: a theory of delinquency', *American Sociological Review*, 2:6 (1957), pp. 664–70.
33 D. Matza, *Delinquency and Drift* (New York: Transaction Publishers, 1990 – original edition 1964).
34 R. S. Agnew, 'Neutralising the impact of crime', *Criminal Justice and Behavior*, 12 (1985), pp. 221–39.
35 For example A. Bandura, 'Selective moral disengagement in the exercise of moral agency', *Journal of Moral Education*, 31:2 (2002), pp. 101–19.
36 Ibid. See also A. Bandura, 'Moral disengagement in the perpetration of inhumanities', *Personality and Social Psychology Review*, 3:3 (1999), pp. 193–209.
37 S. Maruna, *Making Good: How Ex-convicts Reform and Rebuild Their Lives* (Cambridge: American Psychological Association, 2001).
38 Ibid.
39 C. Bollas, *Being a Character: Psychoanalysis and Self-Experience* (London: Routledge, 1993), cited in Cohen, *States of Denial*, p. 26.
40 Cohen, *States of Denial*.
41 For example, J. Hagan, W. Rymond-Richmond & P. Parker, 'The criminology of genocide: the death and rape of Darfur', *Criminology*, 43:3 (2005), pp. 525–62; J. Hagan & W. Rymond-Richmond, 'The collective dynamics of racial dehumanisation and genocidal victimisation in Darfur', *American Sociological Review*, 73 (2008), pp. 875–902.
42 Ibid.
43 C. Lanzmann, *Shoah: The Complete Text of the Acclaimed Holocaust Film* (New York: Da Capo Press, 1995).
44 Ibid.
45 See www.parquedelamemoria.org.ar (accessed 29 January 2014).
46 National Commission on Disappeared People, *Nunca Más: A Report by Argentina's National Commission on Disappeared People* (London: Faber & Faber, 1986).
47 See www.ic-mp.org (accessed 29 January 2014).
48 See www.eaaf.org (accessed 29 January 2014).
49 J. M. Tamarit Summalla, *Historical Memory and Criminal Justice in Spain* (Antwerp: Intersentia, 2013).

50 See www.justice.gov.za/trc (accessed 29 January 2014).
51 S. Neitzel & H. Welzer, *Soldate: On Fighting, Killing and Dying* (London: Simon & Schuster, 2013).
52 See U. Flick, *The SAGE Handbook of Qualitative Data Analysis* (London: Sage, 2013).
53 J. Hagan, *Justice in the Balkans: Prosecuting War Crimes in the Hague Tribunal* (Chicago: University of Chicago Press, 2004).

Bibliography

Agnew, R. S., 'Neutralising the impact of crime', *Criminal Justice and Behavior*, 12 (1985), pp. 221–39

Alexander, L., 'Destructive and self-destructive trends in criminalised society: a study of totalitarianism', *Journal of Criminal Law and Criminology*, 39:5 (1949), pp. 553–64

Alvarez, A., *Governments, Citizens, and Genocide* (Bloomington: Indiana University Press, 2001)

Bandura, A., 'Moral disengagement in the perpetration of inhumanities', *Personality and Social Psychology Review*, 3:3 (1999), pp. 193–209

Bandura, A., 'Selective moral disengagement in the exercise of moral agency', *Journal of Moral Education*, 31:2 (2002), pp. 101–19

Bollas, C., *Being a Character: Psychoanalysis and Self-Experience* (London: Routledge, 1993)

Cohen, S., *States of Denial: Knowing About Atrocities and Suffering* (Cambridge: Polity Press, 2001)

Copes, S. & S. Maruna, 'Excuses, excuses: what have we learned from five decades of neutralisation research?', in M. Tonry (ed.), *Crime and Justice: A Review of Research* (Chicago: University of Chicago Press, 2005), vol. 32, pp. 221–320

Day, L. E. & M. Vandiver, 'Criminology and genocide studies: notes on what might have been and what still could be', *Crime, Law and Social Change*, 34 (2000), pp. 43–59

Elias, N., *The Civilising Process* (Oxford: Blackwell, 2000 – original edition 1939)

Flick, U., *The SAGE Handbook of Qualitative Data Analysis* (London: Sage, 2013)

Freud, S., 'Some psychical consequences of the anatomical distinction between the sexes', *Standard Edition* (London: Hogarth Press, 1925), vol. 19, pp. 248–58

Garland, D., *Peculiar Institution: America's Death Penalty in an Age of Abolition* (New York: Oxford University Press, 2010)

Glueck, E. & S. Glueck, *Physique and Delinquency* (New York: Harper, 1956)

Glueck, S., 'By what tribunal shall war offenders be tried?', *Harvard Law Review*, 56:7 (1943), pp. 1059–89

Glueck, S., *The Nuremburg Trial and Aggressive War* (New York: Knopf, 1946)

Green, P. & T. Ward, *State Crime: Government Violence and Corruption* (London: Pluto Press, 2004)

Hagan, J., *Justice in the Balkans: Prosecuting War Crimes in the Hague Tribunal* (Chicago: University of Chicago Press, 2004)

Hagan, J. & W. Rymond-Richmond, *Darfur and the Crime of Genocide* (New York: Cambridge University Press, 2008)

Hagan, J. & W. Rymond-Richmond, 'The collective dynamics of racial dehumanisation and genocidal victimisation in Darfur', *American Sociological Review*, 73 (2008), pp. 875–902

Hagan, J., W. Rymond-Richmond & P. Parker, 'The criminology of genocide: the death and rape of Darfur', *Criminology*, 43:3 (2005), pp. 525–62

Jenning, W. G., A. R. Piquero & J. M. Reingle, 'On the overlap between victimization and offending: review of the literature', *Aggression and Violent Behavior*, 17 (2012), pp. 16–26

Karstedt, S. & S. Parmentier, 'Introduction to the special issue', *European Journal of Criminology* 9:5 (2012) (special issue, *Atrocity Crimes and Transitional Justice*), pp. 465–7

Kempner, R. M. W., 'Murder by government', *Journal of Criminal Law and Criminology* 38:3 (1948), pp. 235–8

Kittrie, N. N., 'A post mortem of the Eichmann case – the lessons for international law', *Journal of Criminal Law and Criminology*, 55:2 (1964), pp. 16–28

Lanzmann, C., *Shoah: The Complete Text of the Acclaimed Holocaust Film* (New York: Da Capo Press, 1995)

Laufer, W. S., 'The forgotten crime of genocide', in W. S. Laufer & A. Adler (eds), *Advances in Criminological Theory, Volume 8: The Criminology of Criminal Law* (New Brunswick: Transaction Publishers, 1999), pp. 71–82

Loader, I. & R. Sparks, *Public Criminology?* (London: Routledge, 2011)

Lombroso, C., *Criminal Man* (London: Duke University Press, 2006 – original edition 1876)

Maruna, S., *Making Good: How Ex-convicts Reform and Rebuild Their Lives* (Cambridge: American Psychological Association, 2001)

Matza, D., *Delinquency and Drift* (New York: Transaction Publishers, 1990 – original edition 1964)

Morrison, W., *Criminology, Civilisation and the New World Order* (Abingdon: Routledge, 2006)

National Commission on Disappeared People, *Nunca Más: A Report by Argentina's National Commission on Disappeared People* (London: Faber & Faber, 1986)

Neitzel, S. & H. Welzer, *Soldate: On Fighting, Killing and Dying* (London: Simon & Schuster, 2013)

Platt, T., 'Prospects for a radical criminology in the United States', *Crime and Social Justice* 1 (1974), pp. 2–10

Rafter, N., *The Criminal Brain: Understanding Biological Theories of Crime* (New York: New York University Press, 2008)

Savelsberg, J. J., *Crime and Human Rights: Criminology of Genocide and Atrocities* (London: Sage, 2010)

Smeulers, A. & R. Haveman (eds), *Supranational Criminology: Towards a Criminology of International Crimes* (Oxford: Intersentia, 2008)

Spierenburg, P., *Violence and Punishment: Civilising the Body* (Cambridge: Polity Press, 2013)

Sykes, G. M. & D. Matza, 'Techniques of neutralization: a theory of delinquency', *American Sociological Review*, 2:6 (1957), pp. 664–70

Tamarit Summalla, J. M., *Historical Memory and Criminal Justice in Spain* (Antwerp: Intersentia, 2013)

van Kesteren, J., J. van Dijk & P. Mayhew, 'The international crime victim surveys', *International Review of Victimology*, 20 (2014), pp. 49–69

Wetzell, R., *Inventing the Criminal: A History of German Criminology 1880–1945* (Chapel Hill: University of North Carolina Press, 2000)

Yacoubian, G. S., 'The (in)significance of genocidal behaviour to the discipline of criminology', *Crime, Law and Social Change*, 34 (2000), pp. 7–19

5

The disposal of corpses in an ethnicized civil war: Croatia, 1941–45[1]

Alexander Korb

Introduction

In May 1943, an Italian general who was being held prisoner of war was discussing the course of the war with his colleagues. He was describing an incident that had occurred in the territory occupied by Italy in Croatia and, unknown to him, he was overheard by his British supervisors. The incident concerned the recovery of the corpses of murdered Serbs thrown by the perpetrators – Croatian nationalists – into karst caves, which are typical land formations in that area. 'The exhumations were a dreadful task', the general said. 'Nobody could enter the cave because the rotting bodies stank so badly. One man who we lowered down on a rope fainted and we had to pull him out again.'[2] It seems that the soldiers were finally equipped with gas masks.

During the Second World War, up to 45 million people lost their lives.[3] Almost a quarter of them were victims of targeted attacks with the intent to kill and mass murders, rather than armed hostilities. While the death of the victims can be said to have been well researched, many historians consider their task completed once the persecuted individuals have perished. Yet the disposal of bodies in cases of genocide is more than just a field where further research is required; even more important is that the treatment of the dead reveals a great deal about the perpetrators, how they saw themselves, and the approach to and nature of their violence.

The episode described above, which is likely to have occurred in summer 1941 in western Croatia, provides an initial illustration of the complexity of the situation. The Ustaša often threw the bodies of their victims into karst caves, rivers or the sea, or left them on the ground, after having horribly mutilated them. This chapter discusses the massacres carried out by the Ustaša in Croatia during the Second World War. After a brief presentation of the historical background, the massacres carried out by the Ustaša militia and their corpse disposal methods are described. The following section covers the treatment of the dead in the Ustaša camps. The German and Italian reactions to discoveries of the physical traces of the massacres are then discussed. Before the concluding summary, the chapter raises the question of the extent to which the gruesome staging of death, using the corpses of killed opponents, might be part of the communications history of a civil war.

The Ustaša and the Croatian state

The independent state of Croatia was founded in April 1941, following the destruction of Yugoslavia by German troops. Hitler and Mussolini had agreed that an Italian vassal state should be established, to be ruled by the Fascist Croatian Ustaša movement. However, the German Reich and Italy differed on the precise organization of the Croatian state. It was split into two spheres of interest and provided occasion for numerous conflicts between the Axis powers, ranging from the handling of the Ustaša massacres to the question of whether the Jews in the Italian zone should be deported to Auschwitz. The aim of the Ustaša was to convert Croatia into an ethnically homogeneous nation-state, despite the fact that the Catholic Croatian portion of the population was only just over 50 per cent. The Germans supported the Ustaša in the transformation of Croatia into an ethnically homogenized state, and in doing so initially accepted the violent actions of Ustaša militias. What the Germans did not foresee was that, within a very short period, the violent acts of the Ustaša would set in motion a bloody civil war, marking the beginning of both effective opposition and massive counter-violence. The mistakes of German occupation policies and the ravages of the Ustaša transformed the Serbian resistance, and above all the Communist partisans, into successful movements. What had begun as unilateral mass violence on the part of the Ustaša, with their attempt to decimate or annihilate minorities in Croatia, soon developed into a civil war in which three or more parties were fighting against one another, either supported or opposed by the occupation powers, and in which all parties committed war crimes. This observation relating to violence in the context of the civil war should not be seen as equating the atrocities in qualitative terms, for the Ustaša had access to state infrastructure, and could not only dispatch their militia to enemy territory, but could also set up camps and – with the assistance of the Germans – deport tens of thousands of Serbs and Jews. Nevertheless, it can be demonstrated that the rules applying to a dynamic civil war differ from those of traditional genocide. This affected both the murder techniques used and the question of the disposal of the corpses.

The massacres by the Ustaša and the disposal of the dead bodies

A series of massacres accompanied the assumption of power by the Ustaša, in April and May 1941.[4] In June 1941, the use of violence by the Ustaša took on endemic proportions in some regions. In the regions populated by Serbs, especially, there were no Croatian state structures at all, and for this reason it was possible for warlord regimes to become established that were particularly prone to violence; here, the use of violence on the civil population by the militia was part of a battle for regional dominance over local resistance groups, but also against state control from above. In June 1941, the militia began attacking Serbian villages, first in Herzegovina and then in other regions. If villagers were unable to flee beforehand, the band of soldiers marched in and launched massacres, mostly of the male population and sometimes also the female population. The methods of killing varied from one place to another.

What about the way in which they treated the bodies of the dead? Can we assume that a movement engaged in mass murder stops to think about what it is going to do with the corpses of the people it has killed? In general terms, the answer to this question is no. In many cases, the perpetrators made no preparations for the corpses. If they wanted to spare themselves work with the corpses, they simply left the bodies at the location of the massacre and relied on the families or the gendarmerie (the local – though nationally networked – police force) to bury them.[5] Since this did not always occur, fields of stinking corpses were created that polluted the surrounding areas and attracted wild animals.[6] Often the bodies were simply disposed of in nearby rivers.⁷ However, in some cases, the perpetrators hastily buried the dead in mass graves that had been dug in advance, sometimes by the victims themselves; or they blew up the edges of the gullies where the murders had occurred. Villagers often carried out these tasks, too, in forced labour. However, they did not do their work carefully. There were cases of people who were buried while they were still alive, and corpses that were buried either inadequately or incompletely, so that survivors soon began searching for their relatives in the mass graves.⁸

Initially, the Ustaša's victims were unsuspecting and unprepared for the attacks. But from early summer 1941, opposition grew, and with it counter-violence on the part of Serbian and Muslim militia. In general, this meant that the use of violence in the civil war became more multilateral, and the feeling of menace from all sides became more pervasive. Mass murders blurred into paramilitary conflicts in which territories did not usually remain long in the hands of any one warring party. For this reason, the perpetrators often acted in great haste, and in fear of resistance and retaliation they resorted to hit-and-run tactics in which entire villages were set on fire. On occasion they fled the scene of their crimes. Sometimes prisoners were locked in buildings which were then set on fire – but did not always completely burn down. This was the case, for instance, in the Serbian village of Kotorani, which was attacked on 22 August 1941 by a Muslim militia.⁹ On 7 September 1941, a Ustaša mob killed 20 Serbian villagers in the hamlet of Reljevo, near Sarajevo. The prisoners were bound with wire and taken to a house which was then set on fire. Croatian armed forces later found the charred corpses and took photographs.¹⁰

However, the Ustaša practice of throwing the corpses into rivers and caves played a particular role. At the beginning of June 1941, 92 dead Serbs were pulled out of the Vrbas, Vrbanja and Save rivers.¹¹ In mid-June 1941, a Croatian gendarmerie patrol found 14 male corpses that had floated to the estuary of a river. On the first occasions when corpses were washed up or discovered in fields or on the edge of paths, they attracted a great deal of attention. Reporters provided detailed descriptions of the locations, coroners examined the corpses, gendarmes interrogated residents and sought the perpetrators, who were initially unknown.¹² Gendarmerie officers were often the first to find the traces of the massacres and order the disposal of the corpses. In the early stages, in particular, the reports of the gendarmes clearly show that they were very unsure as to how they should interpret the acts of violence by the Ustaša bands. It was still unimaginable that the new Croatian government and its militia had set a mass murder in motion.

The conduct of the militia indicated a certain ambivalence. It appeared to be the simplest solution to throw the corpses into rivers and allow them to float away. In some cases, the imagined destination of the corpses was the sea, a topos that has entered into the contemporary radical right-wing song heritage.[13] At the same time, they put up with the horror disseminated by the floating corpses. In other cases, by contrast, the publicity created by the corpses floating in the rivers was the declared aim of the perpetrators. This is illustrated by an example in which the bodies of a family of four were found tied to one another washed up on land at the end of May 1941 in Bosanska Gradiška. According to a report by the German embassy, a board was fixed to the corpses with the words 'Enjoy your trip to Belgrade'.[14] Thus the corpses served as a means to announce that the Ustaša had assumed power and the Serbs must leave Croatia, dead or alive. The corpses that were washed up were a particular source of horror when they showed signs of abuse or mutilation. Yet the Ustaša bands did not have control over when or where the corpses would be washed up. As a result, the murderers created unanticipated problems for themselves. For instance, in Belgrade, the municipal river baths had to be closed due to the fear of an epidemic, since the Save was deemed to be contaminated. The German authorities in Serbia were anyway very ill-disposed towards the activities of the Ustaša in neighbouring Croatia, and were keen for the situation in Serbia to calm down. Corpses were even occasionally washed up in distant Romania.[15] In der Neretva, clusters of bound corpses obstructed shipping and impaired relations with the Italians, into whose territory the corpses eventually floated.[16] In view of these consequences it is hardly surprising that the practice of throwing corpses into rivers or leaving them at the place of the massacre was a source of abhorrence and provoked massive protests.

An additional special form of violence on the part of the Ustaša became established in the western Croatian karst areas. Here, perpetrators developed the practice of disposing of their victims' bodies by throwing them into the crevices of the widespread karst caves. The great advantages of doing this were that the mass murders could be denied and the troublesome disposal of the corpses was no longer necessary. The numerous karst fissures in western Croatia, which are so typical in the Dinaric Alps, proved suitable for this purpose. Jules Verne described the Dalmatian cave as a 'broad and deep crevice whose steep walls ... fall straight down into the depths. No steps are evident with the help of which one might climb up or down. In other words, we have an abyss before us, the sight of which attracts and captivates us, and which will certainly return to us nothing of that which we throw into it.'[17] The Ustaša militia frequently shot their victims or battered them to death on the edge of such fissures and then pushed them into the depths. Sometimes they threw in hand grenades after the bodies or blew up the entrances to the caves. The first record of this relates to massacres carried out on 3 and 7 June 1941 in the districts of Trebinje and Ljubinje, which were mainly populated by Serbs.[18] Groups of Ustaša militia sent from Zagreb had carried out mass arrests among the local Serbian population. They held the prisoners for a few days, then released a small number of them and apparently decided to kill the remainder. In both instances, they determined to do this during the night. They bound the prisoners, in each case more than 100 people, covered their eyes and took them – by foot or truck – close to the entrance to the caves they deemed suitable for the mass murder. There they bound the men together in small groups, using wire, led them to the edge of the cliff, hit them and fired at them and pushed the severely injured and dead into the depths.[19] While the first massacre went smoothly, from the point of view of the perpetrators, a panic arose among either the perpetrators (a kind of 'forward panic') or the victims on the occasion of the second act of violence (7 June) and this resulted in the escape of up to 50 prisoners.[20] Within a very short period of time, the entire area was informed about the massacre. It soon got around that some of the victims had survived the plunge into the depths. Since, meanwhile, the perpetrators had withdrawn from the scene of the crime near the village of Korita, a group of armed Serbian farmers secured the entry to the cave and, with considerable difficulty, rescued the injured survivors, who received medical aid and were then taken to safe villages or across the border to neighbouring Montenegro. Immediately after the massacres, the Serbian population revolted against the Ustaša.

These two massacres were the first in a long series of slaughters in which Ustaša militia killed Serbian prisoners in karst caves, with their local knowledge proving helpful to them in the process. In at least one instance, the violence was somewhat institutionalized, since a driveway was said to have been constructed to a cave for the specific purpose of facilitating the transportation of the people destined to be killed.[21] Eventually, the other warring parties also got used to throwing corpses in caves. In the second half of the war, Communist partisans are said to have pushed numerous Fascist collaborators into the karst crevices, and the Četnici also made use of this method.[22] On the Italian side, the practice was described in the *foibe*, a narrative with a mystical character telling of victims who, apparently, were mainly Italians.

However, the fact that the corpses vanished into the earth did not mean that the bodies disappeared altogether. Sometimes subterranean rivers flushed them back to the surface,[23] or else the mass graves were discovered – as is still happening nowadays in Slovenia and Croatia.[24] Above all, however, powerful and bloodcurdling myths emerged about the murders in the karsts. For example, it was said that so-called crevice women (*jamarice*) had survived the plunge into the gullies, were living from the food that shepherds occasionally threw down there and had even given birth to children.[25]

Why did the perpetrators resort to throwing corpses into fissures? In Italian historiography, it has been suggested that this was a typical southern Slav violent practice with a ritual character.[26] However, the reasons for this specific approach to killing and corpse disposal in the karst territories are probably related to the form of the landscape rather than the culture of the region and its inhabitants. The murdered victims were pushed into the caves simply because they were there. Nonetheless, one possible specific reason is worth mentioning. With regard to the Communist partisans who threw their opponents into the caves, the historian Rolf Wörsdörfer conjectures that it was also 'the fear of the grief of the enemy, of the extended Serbian Orthodox burial ritual and the suggestive power of the mourning women which persuaded the partisan groups to dispose of the bodies of opponents they had shot'.[27] This may also have played a role for the Ustaša. Furthermore, apart from the practical advantages for the perpetrators, the disappearance of the bodies also represented a threat to the living, which was possibly more effective since it was more covert than the murders, which could be reconstructed and imagined on the basis of rediscovered corpses.

Mass murders in camps

This brings us to the question of how the Ustaša dealt with the corpses of people whom they murdered in their permanent establishments, particularly in camps. While Serbs were the primary victim group of the massacres, as discussed above, mass killings in the camps affected Serbs, Gypsies and Jews equally. It seems, however, that the killers made no distinction between the groups when it came to the treatment of the corpses. Hence when talking about victims of massacres in camps, we are discussing Serbs, Gypsies and Jews.

We need to distinguish between temporary camps and those which were larger and existed for years, in particular the Jasenovac camp. In the former, corpse disposal practices often resembled those of the mobile militia who had carried out massacres of Serbian villagers. Close to the western Croatian town of Gospić there was a group of camps in the summer of 1941 in which the Ustaša interned and murdered Serbian and Jewish prisoners. One of these camps was located on the Mediterranean island of Pag and another close to a hamlet called Jadovno in the coastal mountains. In neither camp had any buildings, such as crematoria, been constructed. Here, the question is whether we can demonstrate that the Ustaša planned the mass murder in advance, or whether it was not, rather, mounting brutality which led to the security guards massacring a large number of the prisoners. Another question in this respect is whether, if the slaughter had been planned in advance, a relatively small, rocky island in the Adriatic could be regarded as suitable for mass murder.

A few weeks after the initial establishment of internment camps in Jadovno and on Pag, the Ustaša security guards there began mass executions of prisoners. The security guards killed hundreds of the prisoners taken to Pag, often immediately after their arrival.[28] They threw many of the corpses into the sea,[29] a technique of mass murder, or corpse disposal, that had been used by other mass murder regimes such as the Ottoman Empire and the Argentine juntas, although the Ustaša did not transport victims out to sea but simply threw them directly off the cliffs into the water. When Italian troops marched into western Croatia in August 1941, the perpetrators panicked, disbanded the camp and killed all the prisoners they could not evacuate from the island. They were, though, unable to dispose of all the corpses in time. When they marched in, the Italian troops were faced with a horrific sight. They found about 800 corpses, which they incinerated.[30] In Jadovno, too, the Italians began recovering the corpses that had been thrown into the karst fissures, although this task proved to be much more difficult. In the area of the camp there are numerous karst caves, some of them up to fifty metres deep.[31] In the years after the war, a number of mass graves were investigated, but some of the crime scenes were never found.

In the more permanent camps, the Ustaša had to adopt a more methodological approach to the disposal of corpses. This applied above all to Jasenovac. Here, too, there were cases where the corpses were thrown into the Save river, but this would not have been sufficient to dispose of all the corpses of those murdered in the camp. The marshy land around the camp, the repeated flooding in the camp and the long frost during the winter made it difficult to construct mass graves, although this was necessary due to the high mortality of the prisoners and the ongoing mass killings. In the winter of 1941–42, the situation in Jasenovac was hellish. Emaciated corpses were piled up in heaps in the open air. Humidity, cramped conditions and thoughtless disposal of the dead led to the outbreak of a typhus epidemic, which further reduced the chances of survival for the prisoners. It was in this situation, in mid-November 1941, that the mass killings of prisoners occurred.[32] However, this created more problems for the camp administration because they could no longer cope with the disposal of the prisoners who had died or been murdered.[33] Since the corpses could not be buried in the frozen earth, they were instead sunk in the Save river.[34]

The question arises as to whether the failure of the perpetrators to dispose of the corpses of their victims also resulted in delays in the murder procedures themselves, as was sometimes the case when the crematoria in the Nazi extermination camps broke down.[35] For instance, Croatian authors have claimed that the mass murders of the Gypsies were postponed from winter to summer 1942 because the ground was frozen and it was not possible to bury the corpses.[36] Apart from the fact that there is no documentary proof for such speculations, they make the assumption that the perpetrators had a coherent extermination programme which they worked through systematically, putting it aside when they encountered difficulties, and resuming it later. No empirical evidence can be provided for this assumption either.

As a reaction to the catastrophe that it had caused, the camp administration attempted to transfer the death zone to the Bosnian side of the Save river, the location of a number of 'killing fields' where mass murders had been carried out since 1942, and where the victims were buried in a very makeshift way in damp ground. Prisoner units were specially created to dispose of the corpses.[37] Later on, a crematorium was built in Jasenovac for the cremation of corpses. However, according to witness reports this was very prone to breakdown and seldom in operation. The disposal of corpses therefore remained a problem until the camp was disbanded.[38] After the war, members of a Yugoslav commission of investigation exhumed numerous bodies in the area of Jasenovac and from the courses of the local rivers.[39]

German and Italian reactions

Because the Ustaša repeatedly left behind unburied corpses of people they had murdered, either intentionally or through carelessness, there were recurring conflicts with the powers whose attention was drawn to the corpses. This applied first and foremost to the Italian occupying forces, but also, to a certain extent, to the Germans. In this connection, scenes occurred such as that described at the beginning of this chapter. The background to this was the complex relationship of the Ustaša with their allies – extremely tense relations in the case of the Italians and an allegiance coloured by mistrust in the case of the Germans – and a fight to the death with their Communist and Nationalist Serbian enemies.

The territory controlled by the Ustaša was very fluid, and as a result they were unable to prevent groups competing with them from gaining access to the locations of the massacres. In August 1941, Croatia and Italy fell out with one another politically, and the Croatian militia were deprived of their power in the Italian sphere of interest in western Croatia, in other words, precisely the area where the Ustaša had previously carried out numerous mass murders. From then on, the Italian army placed greater emphasis on an alliance with the Nationalist Serbian elites. One foundation of this alliance was an arrangement that the people murdered by the Ustaša be respectfully buried. The Italian army therefore organized the recovery of corpses at dozens of locations where massacres had taken place and conducted targeted searches of the karst territories.[40] They went even further, questioning the residents of the surrounding communities and documenting the mass murders.[41] In the vicinity of the Herzegovinian town of Trebinje, for instance, thirteen corpses were recovered on 6 October 1941 – an operation which took an entire day. The bodies were taken by truck to the Serb-Orthodox cemetery of the town and ceremonially buried, to the sound of loud and continuous ringing of the bells. The population took part in large numbers. The burial of 140 corpses in November in Nevisinje followed a similar procedure.

The Croatian gendarmes, who, unlike the Ustaša, had not been driven out of the Italian occupied territory, reported on the events. They disliked the partisan conduct of the Italians – Italian officers, for instance, laid wreaths on the graves – as well as the fact that Croatians were forbidden to attend the ceremony and were thereby being collectively branded as perpetrators. Nevertheless, there were also cases in which the Croatian gendarmerie was ordered to attend exhumations, and this, just as much, was tantamount to a public humiliation.[42] The fear was that the Italian side was attempting to incite people in a targeted way against the Croatian state and was forging an anti-Croatian alliance over the graves of the dead.[43] The Croatian gendarmes were not completely off the mark with their criticism, since the burial ceremonies were cleverly staged as celebrations of Serbian–Italian brotherhood, which both sides were able to exploit politically for their own ends. Thus the Italian military police, the *carabinieri*, used the issue for building the trust of the Serbian population, for instance by visiting Serbian households to inform them when relatives had been killed.[44] Even shortly after the mass murders, some of the entrances to the caves had become places of commemoration, where the dead were remembered and people swore to take up the fight against the Ustaša regime.

The Germans had more difficulties dealing with the locations of the mass murders carried out by their Ustaša partners. Due to strategic alliance considerations, the Germans' reaction was reserved despite their outrage at the massacres. In general terms, they attempted to guide Ustaša policies of persecuting Serbs into 'sensible' channels, prevent mass murders outside the camps and, above all, to rein in public violence.[45] 'More blatant cases' were to be subjected to investigation by the Wehrmacht but the troops were not to intervene.[46] Consequently, German criticism was particularly noisy in cases where the Ustaša made use of gruesome killing methods. However, since the protests were supposed to be submitted through diplomatic channels, cases in which Wehrmacht commanders intervened directly on their own initiative against mass murders remained the exception. If this did occur, however, the German procedure differed little from that employed in the case of the Italians. As early as spring 1941, a Wehrmacht lieutenant ordered that some forty perpetrators be arrested following one of the first Ustaša massacres in Gudovac, and had the corpses, which had been hastily buried in a pit, exhumed and buried. However, the prisoners were released again as a result of political pressure.[47] When the Ustaša carried out a particularly horrific massacre during the night of 23 October 1942 in the village of Palančište near Prijedor, in which some 300 men, women and children were killed with axes and knives, and where the perpetrators also defiled the bodies of the dead, the Wehrmacht ordered that the perpetrators be sought and arrested.[48] The German field gendarmerie and the Croatian gendarmerie carried out the exhumation together.[49] In the case of a massacre in Kukunjevac in October 1942, German soldiers searched for a mass grave with the aid of search dogs. Once they found the grave, which had been partially left open, they sealed it properly.[50] Whether the Wehrmacht officers on the spot intervened against violent actions or not was a matter for their own initiative and determination. None of their supervisors stood in their way. No sanctions were to be expected. On the contrary, a certain pride tends to shine through in army reports in instances where German soldiers showed Ustaša their limits. Nevertheless, this was not in line with German policy, which is why the interventions were no more than individual cases. And as the civil war went on, and the adversaries dug their claws ever more deeply into one another, it became increasingly difficult to guide the violence in any way.

Demonstrative violence – a means of communication

To a greater extent than in a conventional war, and more, too, than in cases of asymmetrical use of violence, where the perpetrators have a monopoly over violence, the participants in a civil war communicate by trying to shock a sense of fear into their opponents and to spread horror among the enemy civil population.[51] It was obvious that the opposing side would respond to the way in which the corpses had been left behind. Mountains of corpses or individual human bodies thus contained explicit or implicit messages to opponents. Nevertheless, it would be wrong to see messages in all aspects of violent activities, and it is important to comprehend the ambivalence of this morbid legacy since, in the first instance, the horrific violent acts were, above all, an expression of the whipped up hatred and passions in an emotional civil war that people regarded as existential. In many areas, it was hardly possible to put a stop to the Ustaša attacks on the Serbian civil population. In addition, there was, however, an instrumental level to many violent acts that needs to be deciphered.

Thus it was that the Ustaša, in their ideological hatred, were unable to desist from attacks on the Serbian population. At the same time, this conformed to their strategy of preventing any stabilization of the situation wherever possible, since they had set themselves up well in their system of warlord dominions. Pacification of their battle territory would have put an end to their highway robbery and they might also have been called to account for their deeds. For this reason, too, they torpedoed all attempts to pacify Croatia. Here are two examples that illustrate this strategy. In order to halt the insurgency, the authorities, supported by the Wehrmacht, repeatedly called upon the civil population to return to their villages and promised them exemption from punishment as well as personal safety and the safety of their property in return. In this situation, all the militia had to do was to attack individual returning villagers – and then this laboriously established trust would be destroyed in one fell swoop.[52] In one instance in Bosanska Krupa, '14 Serbian insurgents who had laid down their weapons were literally slaughtered with knives by Ustaše'.[53] When negotiators for the Četnici and the Croatian authorities attempted, in spring 1942, to negotiate a cease-fire, a Ustaša militia again intervened, surrounding the location where the negotiations were being conducted with some 100 armed men, killing a Serb and then having his severed head carried on a pole through the town. As might be expected, this resulted in an immediate breakdown in the negotiations.[54] Thus, murders were particularly brutal in cases where the militia wished to indicate to the Serbian population that peaceful coexistence was impossible. This message could be directed at people returning home, negotiators or Serbian converts to Catholicism. However, the most gruesome was the violence against people who, from the point of view of the Ustaša, represented everything they were fighting against. The perpetrators invested much time, energy and strength in many of the crimes against Orthodox priests or certain representatives of the Serbian resistance, and they did so in a manner that is reminiscent of ritual murder. Before killing their victims, they often abused them in the most gruesome manner. This included setting fire to beards, gouging out eyes, cutting off body members, noses, ears and tongues and slashing open their bodies.[55] Tools such as knives, wooden wedges, hammers and axes were used. The emotional closeness of the perpetrators to their victims is evident in view of the lack of distance in their methods of killing. In such cases, exhibiting body members documented, as it were, the completion of the deed.

Finally, the militia carried out numerous acts of sexual violence. Mass rape is typically an aspect of the violence in a civil war. The male dominance of the militia, the unlimited and general brutality and the blurring of borders between combatants and the civil population allow soldiers to commit acts in times of war they could not engage in during peacetime.[56] Here it is of interest to note that the murderers deliberately left the corpses of the women they had raped either naked or placed in specific positions, to transmit to their (male) war opponents the message that they were unable to protect their women. This also related explicitly to pregnant women, as the Wehrmacht reported in June 1942 after they had found several mutilated corpses of murdered Serb women.[57]

Summary

We obtained the picture of a complex situation in which several parties in Croatia fought one another over a period of years. The trigger for both the intercommunal violence and the civil war was the mass murders by the Ustaša, who carried out these massacres in their attempt to assume dominance over a multi-ethnic territory, push through their ethnocratic regime and decimate the Serbian population. However, this mass violence was characterized by regional variations, different kinds of action on the part of the differing perpetrator groups and varying forms of violence. Overall, there was little planning or system in the acts of violence, even if the Ustaša probably achieved their terrorist goals, since they provoked panic in the Serbian settlement area, leading to expulsions and a mass flight of Serbs out of Croatia.

The unsystematic procedures of the Ustaša militia were also reflected in their treatment of the dead. Massacres in rural areas followed very variable patterns. Sometimes corpses were disposed of but at other times not. Thus, by comparison with the mass murders carried out by the German Security Police and Security Service task forces in the occupied Soviet Union, the procedures were not very systematic. That applies to the treatment of the human remains of the murdered as well. In their eastern territories, the Germans desperately tried to cover up all traces of the genocide they had committed. Once the Soviet troops started advancing and liberating territories where mass executions had taken place, a task force ('Action 1005') was put in charge to destroy the evidence, to exhume mass graves and to incinerate the corpses. The Special Command 4a unit under SS-Standartenführer Blobel developed a whole range of techniques for the disposal of corpses.

In Croatia, nothing like that happened. The Germans framed the atrocities in Croatia in terms of an unavoidable civil war that had resulted from ancient hatreds, and less in terms of a unilateral genocide with a clear group of perpetrators on the one hand and victims on the other. The Germans did not feel responsible for the Ustaša genocide and felt they had had nothing to hide. Moreover, the Ustaša mass murder of Serbs, Jews and Gypsies was public knowledge.[58] They did, however, destroy traces of the mass murder of Jews they had committed in Serbia.[59] Interestingly, Paul Blobel was transferred to Croatia in October 1944. But there he was not responsible for 'unearthing' any longer. Instead, he headed an anti-partisan unit.

In terms of the lack of systematic fashion of mass murder, much the same applies to the Ustaša camps. The name often given to Jasenovac, 'Auschwitz of the Balkan Peninsular', hides more than it reveals,[60] since – more frequently still than in the German extermination camps – mass murder in the Ustaša camps was characterized by a momentum that was hard to rein in, by loss of control and mass deaths that were often, but not always, intended. Thus it is hardly astonishing that, when it came to the disposal of corpses, the security guards ultimately lost control and that attempts to dispose of corpses in the camp were erratic.

When the armed uprisings against the Ustaša regime began in the summer of 1941, the nature of the violence altered. Although the greatest violence, in quantitative terms, and the most systematic and brutal, in qualitative terms, continued to originate from the Ustaša, from then on the Ustaša were no longer the only group carrying out violent acts, since the country slid into a civil war in which all sides were responsible for violence. The civil war parties were now fighting an existential battle against one another in which, in their view, the only outcome could be victory or defeat. This explains the emotional content of the violence and some of the symbolic subtext. More than previously, the hostile groups were communicating with each another through their acts of murder. In this respect, the Ustaša attained mastery since they had a vested interest in stoking up the ethnicized civil war, which was helping to legitimize the existence of the militia. They wanted to make sure that a multi-ethnic Yugoslav society could never come into existence again. By defiling corpses and exhibiting the bodies, they wished to show their opponents that peaceful coexistence would never again return.

Notes

1 The text of this chapter was translated from the author's German by Cadenza Academic Translations.
2 Taken from a transcript of the overheard remarks of an Italian general held as a prisoner of war. BRIG 33, 26 May 1943, UK National Archives, w.o. 38/2154, pp. 1-3.
3 J. Echternkamp, *Die 101 wichtigsten Fragen: Der Zweite Weltkrieg* (Munich: Beck, 2010), p. 139.
4 See A. Korb, *Im Schatten des Weltkriegs: Massengewalt der Ustaša gegen Serben, Juden und Roma in Kroatien 1941-1945* (Hamburg: Hamburg Edition, 2013).
5 This occurred after a massacre in Sekulinci, Slavonia, in the Papuk mountains in February 1942. See German Embassy Zagreb (DGA), Report (appendix 2c), 26 October 1942, German Federal Military Archives (henceforth BA-MA), RH 31 III/7. Also, after many massacres, the bodies were scattered over a wide area, especially when the Ustaša had been pursuing fugitives. See V. Dedijer, *The War Diaries of Vladimir Dedijer* (Ann Arbor: University of Michigan Press, 1990), p. 270.
6 Report by the 3rd Ustaša platoon of the 1st Infantry Battalion, July 1941, printed in *Borbe u Bosni i Hercegovini 1941 god.: Knjiga 1*, Zbornik dokumenata i podataka o narodnooslobodilačkom ratu jugoslovenskih naroda, vol. 4 (Belgrade: Vojnoistorijski Institut Jugoslovenske Armije, 1951). See also Arthur Häffner to DGiA, 23 June 1941, BA-MA, RH 31 III/13, p. 10.
7 Interview with Miloš Despot from Bijeljina, US Holocaust Memorial Museum (henceforth USHMM) Archives RG-50.468/10, Tape 1. See also P. Broucek (ed.), *Deutscher Bevollmächtigter General in Kroatien und Zeuge des Untergangs des 'Tausendjährigen Reiches'. Ein General im Zwielicht. Edmund Glaise von Horstenau* (Vienna: Böhlau, 1988), p. 168.
8 The 1st Gendarmerie Division related in a report dated 16 August 1941 to the RAVSIGUR how the surviving Serbian population coped with the consequences of the mass murder. Serbian Military Archives (henceforth AVII), NDH/145, 2/1.
9 3rd HOP to RAVSIGUR, 28 August 1941, AVII, NDH/145, 6/43. The name of the village was Kotor or Kotorani.
10 Interrogation by Muja Sadžak, gendarmerie commander in Sarajevo, 30 September 1941, AVII, NDH/150a, 2/28.
11 DGA, Report (appendix 2), 26 October 1942, BA-MA, RH 31 III/7, without running number. Already at the end of May 1941, the corpse of the Orthodox bishop of Banja Luka, Platon, was found at the confluence of the two rivers.
12 Gendarmerie post Ilidža to 4th HOP, Report no. 207, 25 May 1941, AVII, NDH 143B, 41/1-3, printed in S. Vukčević, (ed.), *Zločini Nezavisne Države Hrvatske, 1941-1945*, Zločini na jugoslovenskim prostorima u prvom i drugom svetskom ratu: Zbornik dokumenata 1 (Belgrade: Vojnoistorijski institut, 1993), p. 57, doc. 34, as well as gendarmerie Zenica to 4th HOP, 18 June 1941, AVII, NDH/143, 1/18-1.

13 Rock band Thompson makes reference to this topos, possibly referring to contemporary songs.
14 See Serbian Eastern Orthodox Diocese of the United States of America and Canada (ed.), *Martyrdom of the Serbs: Persecutions of the Serbian Orthodox Church and Massacre of the Serbian People* (Chicago: Palandech's Press, 1943).
15 American Joint Distribution Committee Belgrade report on washed up corpses, 13 March 1946, in Yad Vashem Archives (YVA), O.10/11, Bl. 4 and YVA, O.10/3-1-5. In the 1990s, the story and even possibly the practice was reinstated. See J. B. Allcock, *Explaining Yugoslavia* (New York: Columbia University Press, 2000), p. 382.
16 See S. Kvesić, *Dalmacija u narodnooslobodilačkoj borbi* (Split: Vojna Štamparia, 1979), p. 79; J. Steinberg, *All or Nothing: The Axis and the Holocaust 1941–1943* (London: Routledge, 1990), p. 49.
17 Quoted in J. Strutz (ed.), *Dalmatien* (Klagenfurt: Europa erlesen – Wieser Verlag, 1998), p. 61. See also R. Wörsdörfer, *Krisenherd Adria 1915–1955: Konstruktion und Artikulation des Nationalen im italienisch-jugoslawischen Grenzraum* (Paderborn: Ferdinand Schöningh Verlag, 2004), p. 477, who discusses the link between violence and landscape forms in relation to the karst.
18 The description of the massacre of Korita is based on T. Dulić, *Utopias of Nation: Local Mass Killing in Bosnia and Herzegovina, 1941–42*, Acta Universitatis Upsaliensis vol. 218 (Uppsala: Uppsala University Press, 2005), p. 124. See also J. Tomasevich, *War and Revolution in Yugoslavia, 1941–1945: Occupation and Collaboration* (Stanford: Stanford University Press, 2001), p. 938; B. Kovačević & S. Skoko, 'Junski ustanak u Hercegovini 1941. godine' ('The June 1941 uprising in Hercegovina'), in *Istorija radničkog pokreta: Zbornik radova I* (Belgrade: Institut za izučavanje radničkog pokreta, 1965), p. 107.
19 The statements are to be found in the Archives of Serbia and in the Archives of Yugoslavia and some of them have been published. See M. Bjelica, 'Zapisi sa koritske jame', in S. Kovačević (ed.), *Hercegovina u NOB* (Belgrade: Vojnoizdavački i Novinski Centar, 1986); V. Dedijer & A. Miletić (eds), *Proterivanje Srba sa ognjišta 1941–1944: Svedočanstva* (Belgrade: Prosveta, 1989), p. 155.
20 Dulić, *Utopias of Nation*, pp. 136ff. For the massacre at Ljubinje see S. Radić, *Lubinje i Popovo polje, 1941–1945* (Lubinje: Kultura, 1969), p. 2217.
21 For reports of this kind about a cave near the village of Boričevac on the Bosnian–Croatian border, not far from Kulen Vakuf, see R. Pilipović, 'Bosanska krajina u Drugom svetskom ratu: U ogledalu sudbine Srpske pravoslavne crkve', at http://pravoslavlje.spc.rs/broj/978/tekst/bosanska-krajina-u-drugom-svetskom-ratu/print/lat (accessed 3 December 2013).
22 On partisans see K.-P. Schwarz, 'Auch Norma lebte noch', *Frankfurter Allgemeine Zeitung*, 27 March 2010, p. 3; for the Četnici see J. Jurjević, *Pogrom u Krnjeuši 9. i 10. kolovoza 1941* (Zagreb: Vikarijat Banjalučke biskupije, 1999).

An ethnicized civil war: Croatia   123

23 M. Djilas, *Der Krieg der Partisanen: Jugoslawien 1941–1945* (Vienna: Molden Verlag, 1978), p. 126. [In English: *Wartime* (New York: Harcourt, 1980)]
24 See for example *Der Spiegel* online, 'Einestages, Rätsel der verschwundenen Division', http://einestages.spiegel.de/static/topicalbum background/3931/1/raetsel_der_verschwundenen_division.html (accessed 31 May 2012).
25 N. Sremac, *Zapisi sa drugog zasjedanja ANVOJ-a* (Zagreb: Znanje, 1964), p. 43.
26 See Wörsdörfer, *Krisenherd Adria*, pp. 483, 502.
27 Ibid., pp. 483, 502.
28 N. Lengel-Krizman & M. Sobolevski, 'Hapšenje 165 omladinaca u Zagrebu u svibnju 1941. g', *Novi Omanut*, 31 (1998), pp. 7–9; M. Peršen, *Ustaški logori* (Zagreb: Globus, 1990), p. 84; for the report of a survivor see the statement by Bozo Švarc, no. 571/45, 17 July 1945, Croatian State Archives (henceforth HAD), ZKRZ-GUZ 2235/6-45, k. 11. See also B. Švarc, 'Kako sam preživio', *Ha-kol*, 69–70 (2001), pp. 5ff.
29 10th military post to Command 2nd Italian army, 1 August 1941, YVA, O.10/64, Bl. 3.
30 See M. Shelah, *Heshbon Damim: Hatzalat Yehude Croatiah al yedey ha-italkim, 1941–1943* (Tel Aviv: Moreshet, 1986), p. 35; I. Goldstein & S. Goldstein, *Holokaust u Zagrebu* (Zagreb: Novi Liber, 2001), p. 292. Non-verifiable extracts from a report by an Italian army commission are printed in A. Zemljar, *Haron i Sudbine: Ustaški koncentracioni logori Slana i Metajna na ostrvu Pagu – 1941* (Belgrade: Četvrti jul, 1988), p. 222, at www.jadovno.com/ originalni-dokumenti-talijanske-vojno-sanitetske-sluzbe.html (accessed 31 May 2012). See also Peršen, *Ustaški logori*, p. 101. For Croatian reports on the Italian procedure see Zap. 1. puk. an Ravsigur, 21 September 1941, AVII, NDH/152, 5/43.
31 According to Zatezalo, the perpetrators made the scene of the crime unrecognizable by pouring concrete into the karst caves. See Đ. Zatezalo, *Jadovno: Kompleks ustaških logora 1941* (Belgrade: Muzej žrtava genocida, 2007), vol. 1, p. 738. However, it is doubtful whether they went to so much trouble in view of the imminent Italian occupation.
32 See recollections of Albert Maestro, printed in D. Sindik (ed.), *Sećanja Jevreja na logor Jasenovac* (Belgrade: Savez jevrejskih opština Jugoslavije, 1972), p. 122.
33 See N. Mataušić (ed.) (with N. Jovičić), *Jasenovac Concentration Camp: Exhibition About the Beginning of the Camp System, August 1941–February 1942* (Zagreb: Biblioteka Kameni Cvijet, 2003), p. 35. See also recollections of Jakov Kabiljo and Albert Maestro, printed in Sindik, *Sećanja Jevreja*, pp. 87, 123; the latter reports that the unit to which he belonged buried 1,200 corpses. See also Peršen, *Ustaški logori*, p. 139.
34 See recollections of Jakov Kabiljo, in Sindik, *Sećanja Jevreja*, p. 87.
35 R. J. van Pelt, 'Auschwitz', in G. Morsch, B. Perz & A. Ley (eds), *Neue Studien zu nationalsozialistischen Massentötungen durch Giftgas: Historische Bedeutung, technische Entwicklung, revisionistische Leugnung* (Berlin: Metropol Verlag, 2011).

36 N. Lengel-Krizman, 'Genocide carried out on the Roma: Jasenovac 1942', in Jasenovac Memorial Area Public Institution (ed.), *Jasenovac Memorial Site: Catalogue* (Jasenovac: Biblioteka Kameni Cvijet, 2006), p. 162.
37 See Goldstein & Goldstein, *Holokaust u Zagrebu*, p. 317.
38 See Dulić, *Utopias of Nation*, p. 277.
39 USHMM, Photograph #46689.
40 See report by the Croatian gendarmerie post at Široka Kula, 3 September 1941, s. Zapovjednictvo OK Gospić to Grupa Generala Lukica kod 2. Talianske Armate, 3 September 1941, AVII, NDH/67, 3/20-1.
41 VOZ Mostar to the military office of Poglavnik, 18 September 1942, AVII, NDH/229, MHD br. 4628/Taj; and report of the Croatian gendarmerie post at Široka Kula, 3 September 1941, AVII, NDH/67, 3/20-1; and S. Trifković, 'The Ustaša movement and European politics, 1929–1945', unpublished dissertation, University of Southampton (1990), p. 223. In some cases, petrol was poured on the corpses by the Italian army and they were incinerated; see 1st HOP to RAVSIGUR, 21 September 1941, AVII, NDH/152, 5/43.
42 Wing command of gendarmerie Bileća to 4th HOP, 27 November 1941, AVII, NDH/143a, 7/29-1; gendarmerie post Ravno to 4th HOP, 22 September 1941, AVII, NDH/143c, 3/30-1.
43 A large number of reports exist, differing in their detail but consistent in the general tenor. See Commander 4th HOP Sarajevo to Ravsigur, 8 October 1941, AVII, NDH/143a, 4/19-1, and Oruz. Krilno Zap. u Bileci to Zap. 4th HOP, 27 November 1941, AVII, NDH/143a, 7/29-1, and camp report 16–31 August 1942, VOZ to PVU, 10 September 1942; Croatian State Archives, HR HDA 223/30, no. 1180, and gendarmerie post Ravno, 22 September 1941. See also Report by the Ministry of Interior, 7 November 1941. Trifković, 'The Ustaša movement', p. 223.
44 Report by the Ministry of Interior, 7 November 1941, Croatian State Archives, HR HDA 223/30, no. 1180.
45 For the speech on a 'sensible solution to the Serbian problem', see Tomasevich, *War and Revolution*, p. 440.
46 Glaise to the OKW, 10 July 1941, BA-MA, 20-12/454, Fs no. 187/41.
47 See Kasche to AA, 30 April 1941, US National Archives and Records Administration (henceforth NARA) T-120/5787, H301722; Goldstein & Goldstein, *Holokaust u Zagrebu*, p. 94; Tomasevich, *War and Revolution*, p. 398.
48 Report by the 3rd Croatian gendarmerie regiment, 10 October 1942, AVII, NDH/162, 8/14-1.
49 Statement by Banović, AVII, NDH, 44/7-2, 162; Wing commander of gendarmerie Banja Luka to senior state and military posts (circular), 12 November 1942, AVII, NDH/162, 9/27. On the justification of the massacre on the part of the Ustaša as a military exercise, see the report by the 8th Ustaša batallion, AVII, NDH, 4-63, 76.
50 See VOZ to circulation, 23 October 1942, AVII, NDH/75, 4/2-1.
51 See S. Kalyvas, *The Logic of Violence in Civil War* (Cambridge: Cambridge University Press, 2006).

An ethnicized civil war: Croatia 125

52 DGA, Report (appendix 2), 26 October 1942, BA-MA, RH 31 III/7, without running no.
53 Arthur Häffner to DGiA, 27 August 1941, BA-MA, RH 31 III/13, p. 49.
54 4th HOP to VOZ, 4 March 1942, AVII, NDH/75, 3/17-1.
55 The torments mentioned here are based on a DGA record (passed on to the Military Commander, Serbia, 24 June 1941), quoted in Vukčević, *Zločini Nezavisne Države Hrvatske*, p. 137, doc. 76. See also the Wehrmacht, 718. ID, Ia to Kdr.Gen.u.Bef.i.S., passed on to OKW, 9 June 1942, NARA, T-501/250, fr. 1072 et seq.; as well as the report of the Croatian commander of the military border to the military office of Poglavnik of 4 September 1941, Historical Museum of Bosnia and Hercegovina (HM BiH), NDH/1941, no. 92. In the reports of the survivors of the Ustaša massacres inside and outside the camps there are numerous descriptions of boundless and sadistic acts of violence. See for instance E. Berger, *44 mjeseca u Jasenovcu* (Zagreb: Grafički zavod Hrvatske, 1966); M. Kolar-Dimitrijević, 'Sjećanja veterinara Zorka Goluba na trinaest dana boravka u logoru Jasenovac 1942. Godine', *Časopis za Suvremenu Povijest*, 15:2 (1983), pp. 155–76, 175; A. Ciliga, *Sam kroz Europu u ratu, 1939–1945* (Rome: Na Pragu sutrašnjice, 1978), p. 236; Savez Jevrejskih Opština, *Zločini fašističkih okupatora i njihovih pomagača protiv Jevreja u Jugoslaviji* (Belgrade: Association of Jewish Communities in Yugoslavia, 1952), p. 93. See also Broucek, *Deutscher Bevollmächtigter General*, p. 165; V. Kazimirović, *NDH u svetlu nemačkih dokumenata i dnevnika Gleza fon Horstenau, 1941–1944* (Belgrade: Nova knj. Nar. knj., 1987), p. 111. On the use of both blunt and sharp weapons when killing see Arthur Häffner to D.G.i.A., 3 August 1941, BA-MA, RH 31 III/13, Bl. 42; and ZHO to all central posts of the state, the Ustaša and the army, 18 February 1942, AVII, NDH/75, 2/16-1, report no. 431 taj; interview with Miloš Despot from Bijeljina, USHMM RG-50.468/10, Tape 1.
56 See E. von Erdmann,'Vergewaltigung als Kommunikation zwischen Männern: Kontexte und Auseinandersetzung in Publizistik und Literatur', in M. Erstić, S. Kabić & B. Künkel (eds), *Opfer, Beute, Boten der Humanisierung? Zur künstlerischen Rezeption der Überlebensstrategien von Frauen im Bosnienkrieg und im Zweiten Weltkrieg* (Bielefeld: Transcript Verlag, 2012).
57 See Kom.Gen.u.Bef.i.Serbien, Ia, to OKW, 9 June 1942, NARA, T-501/250, fr. 1072, and 718. ID, Ia to Kom.Gen.u.Bef.i.Serbien, 9 June 1942, NARA T-501/250, fr. 1074; in addition, Chief Sipo/SD Belgrad sent a report to the police attaché in Zagreb, Helm – see NARA, T-120/5786, H300761 et seq.
58 Korb, *Im Schatten des Weltkriegs*, pp. 305f.
59 R. B. Birn, 'Austrian higher SS and police leaders and their participation in the Holocaust in the Balkans', *Holocaust and Genocide Studies*, 6:4 (1991), pp. 351–72, at p. 359.
60 V. Dedijer, *Jasenovac – das jugoslawische Auschwitz und der Vatikan* (Freiburg: Ahriman Verlag, 1989).

Bibliography

Allcock, J. B., *Explaining Yugoslavia* (New York: Columbia University Press, 2000)
Berger, E., *44 mjeseca u Jasenovcu* (Zagreb: Grafički zavod Hrvatske, 1966)
Birn, R. B., 'Austrian higher SS and police leaders and their participation in the Holocaust in the Balkans', *Holocaust and Genocide Studies*, 6:4 (1991), pp. 351–72
Bjelica, M., 'Zapisi sa koritske jame', in S. Kovačević (ed.), *Hercegovina u NOB* (Belgrade: Vojnoizdavački i Novinski Centar, 1986), pp. 69–76
Broucek, P. (ed.), *Deutscher Bevollmächtigter General in Kroatien und Zeuge des Untergangs des 'Tausendjährigen Reiches'. Ein General im Zwielicht. Edmund Glaise von Horstenau* (Vienna: Böhlau, 1988), vol. 3
Ciliga, A., *Sam kroz Europu u ratu, 1939–1945* (Rome: Na Pragu Sutrašnjice, 1978)
Dedijer, V., *Jasenovac – das jugoslawische Auschwitz und der Vatikan* (Freiburg: Ahriman Verlag, 1989)
Dedijer, V., *The War Diaries of Vladimir Dedijer* (Ann Arbor: University of Michigan Press, 1990)
Dedijer, V. & A. Miletić (eds), *Proterivanje Srba sa ognjišta 1941–1944: Svedočanstva* (Belgrade: Prosveta, 1989)
Der Spiegel online, 'Einestages, Rätsel der verschwundenen Division', http://einestages.spiegel.de/static/topicalbumbackground/3931/1/raetsel_der_verschwundenen_division.html
Djilas, M., *Der Krieg der Partisanen: Jugoslawien 1941–1945* (Vienna: Molden Verlag, 1978) [in English: *Wartime* (New York: Harcourt, 1980)]
Dulić, T., *Utopias of Nation: Local Mass Killing in Bosnia and Herzegovina, 1941–42*, Acta Universitatis Upsaliensis vol. 218 (Uppsala: Uppsala University Press, 2005)
Echternkamp, J., *Die 101 wichtigsten Fragen: Der Zweite Weltkrieg* (Munich: Beck, 2010)
Erstić, M., S. Kabić & B. Künkel (eds), *Opfer, Beute, Boten der Humanisierung? Zur künstlerischen Rezeption der Überlebensstrategien von Frauen im Bosnienkrieg und im Zweiten Weltkrieg* (Gender Studies) (Bielefeld: Transcript Verlag, 2012)
Goldstein, I. & S. Goldstein, *Holokaust u Zagrebu* (Zagreb: Novi Liber, 2001)
Goldstein, S., *1941: Godina koja se vraća* (Zagreb: Novi Liber, 2007)
Jurjević, J., *Pogrom u Krnjeuši 9. i 10. kolovoza 1941* (Zagreb: Vikarijat Banjalučke Biskupije, 1999)
Kalyvas, S., *The Logic of Violence in Civil War* (Cambridge: Cambridge University Press, 2006)
Kazimirović, V., *NDH u svetlu nemačkih dokumenata i dnevnika Gleza fon Horstenau, 1941–1944* (Belgrade: Nova knj. Nar. knj., 1987)
Kolar-Dimitrijević, M., 'Sjećanja veterinara Zorka Goluba na trinaest dana boravka u logoru Jasenovac 1942. Godine', *Časopis za Suvremenu Povijest*, 15:2 (1983), pp. 155–76

Korb, A., *Im Schatten des Weltkriegs: Massengewalt der Ustaša gegen Serben, Juden und Roma in Kroatien 1941–1945* (Hamburg: Hamburger Edition, 2013)
Kovačević, B. & S. Skoko, 'Junski ustanak u Hercegovini 1941. godine', in *Istorija radničkog pokreta: Zbornik radova I* (Belgrade: Institut za izučavanje radničkog pokreta, 1965)
Kovačević, S. (ed.), *Hercegovina u NOB* (Belgrade: Vojnoizdavački i Novinski Centar, 1986)
Kvesić, S., *Dalmacija u narodnooslobodilačkoj borbi* (Split: Vojna Štamparia, 1979)
Lengel-Krizman, N., 'Genocide carried out on the Roma: Jasenovac 1942', in Jasenovac Memorial Area Public Institution (ed.), *Jasenovac Memorial Site: Catalogue* (Jasenovac: Biblioteka Kameni Cvijet, 2006), pp. 154–81
Lengel-Krizman, N. & M. Sobolevski, 'Hapšenje 165 omladinaca u Zagrebu u svibnju 1941. g', *Novi Omanut*, 31 (1998), pp. 7–9
Mataušić, N. (ed.) (with N. Jovičić), *Jasenovac Concentration Camp: Exhibition About the Beginning of the Camp System, August 1941–February 1942* (Zagreb: Biblioteka Kameni Cvijet, 2003)
Peršen, M., *Ustaški logori* (Zagreb: Globus, 1990)
Pilipović, R., 'Bosanska krajina u Drugom svetskom ratu: U ogledalu sudbine Srpske pravoslavne crkve', at http://pravoslavlje.spc.rs/broj/978/tekst/bosanska-krajina-u-drugom-svetskom-ratu/print/lat
Radić, S., *Lubinje i Popovo polje, 1941–1945* (Lubinje: Kultura, 1969)
Rimay, T. (ed.), *Jasenovac Memorial Site: Catalogue* (Jasenovac: Biblioteka Kameni Cvijet, 2006)
Savez Jevrejskih Opština, *Zločini fašističkih okupatora i njihovih pomagača protiv Jevreja u Jugolaviji* (Belgrade: Association of Jewish Communities in Yugoslavia, 1952)
Schwarz, K.-P., 'Auch Norma lebte noch', *Frankfurter Allgemeine Zeitung*, 27 March 2010, p. 3
Serbian Eastern Orthodox Diocese of the United States of America and Canada (ed.), *Martyrdom of the Serbs: Persecutions of the Serbian Orthodox Church and Massacre of the Serbian People* (Chicago: Palandech's Press, 1943), Documents and reports of the trustworthy United Nations and of eyewitnesses
Shelah, M., *Heshbon Damim: Hatzalat Yehude Croatiah al yedey ha-italkim, 1941–1943* (Tel Aviv: Moreshet, 1986)
Sindik, D. (ed.), *Sećanja Jevreja na logor Jasenovac* (Belgrade: Savez jevrejskih opština Jugoslavije, 1972)
Sremac, N., *Zapisi sa drugog zasjedanja ANVOJ-a* (Zagreb: Znanje, 1964)
Steinberg, J., *All or Nothing: The Axis and the Holocaust 1941–1943* (London: Routledge, 1990)
Strutz, J. (ed.), *Dalmatien* (Klagenfurt: Europa erlesen – Wieser Verlag, 1998)
Švarc, B., 'Kako sam preživio', *Ha-kol*, 69–70 (2001), pp. 5ff.
Tomasevich, J., *War and Revolution in Yugoslavia, 1941–1945: Occupation and Collaboration* (Stanford: Stanford University Press, 2001)

Trifković, S., 'The Ustaša movement and European politics, 1929–1945', unpublished dissertation, University of Southampton (1990)
van Pelt, R. J., 'Auschwitz', in G. Morsch, B. Perz & A. Ley (eds), *Neue Studien zu nationalsozialistischen Massentötungen durch Giftgas: Historische Bedeutung, technische Entwicklung, revisionistische Leugnung* (Berlin: Metropol Verlag, 2011), pp. 196–218
Vojnoistorijski Institut Jugoslovenske Armije, *Borbe u Bosni i Hercegovini 1941 god.: Knjiga 1*, Zbornik dokumenata i podataka o narodnooslobodilačkom ratu jugoslovenskih naroda, vol. 4 (Belgrade: Vojnoistorijski Institut Jugoslovenske Armije, 1951)
von Erdmann, E., 'Vergewaltigung als Kommunikation zwischen Männern: Kontexte und Auseinandersetzung in Publizistik und Literatur', in M. Erstić, S. Kabić & B. Künkel (eds), *Opfer, Beute, Boten der Humanisierung? Zur künstlerischen Rezeption der Überlebensstrategien von Frauen im Bosnienkrieg und im Zweiten Weltkrieg* (Bielefeld: Transcript Verlag, 2012), pp. 13–38
Vukčević, S. (ed.), *Zločini Nezavisne Države Hrvatske, 1941–1945*, Zločini na jugoslovenskim prostorima u prvom i drugom svetskom ratu: Zbornik dokumenata 1 (Belgrade: Vojnoistorijski institut, 1993)
Wörsdörfer, R., *Krisenherd Adria 1915–1955: Konstruktion und Artikulation des Nationalen im italienisch-jugoslawischen Grenzraum* (Paderborn: Ferdinand Schöningh Verlag, 2004)
Zatezalo, Đ., *Jadovno: Kompleks ustaških logora 1941* (Belgrade: Muzej žrtava genocida, 2007), vol. 1
Zemljar, A., *Haron i Sudbine: Ustaški koncentracioni logori Slana i Metajna na ostrvu Pagu – 1941* (Belgrade: Četvrti jul, 1988)

Archives

Croatian State Archives, Zagreb (HDA)
German Federal Military Archives, Freiburg i.B. (BA-MA)
Historical Museum of Bosnia and Hercegovina, Sarajevo (HM BiH)
Serbian Military Archives, Belgrade (AVII)
UK National Archives, Kew
US Holocaust Memorial Museum, Washington, DC (USHMM)
US National Archives and Records Administration, College Park, MD (NARA)
Yad Vashem Archives, Jerusalem (YVA)

6

Renationalizing bodies? The French search mission for the corpses of deportees in Germany, 1946–58[1]

Jean-Marc Dreyfus

Introduction

Corpses are not a research subject that a historian would normally choose, and less still corpses en masse. Whether approaches to mass violence are of political, social or cultural history, the historical analysis of societies tends to focus on the living, and corpses are discussed only in terms of a social group's structure in relation to death, the social definition of which can be addressed only through a detailed cultural history.[2] While the study of funerary rites has always been central in anthropology for example, this has not often been the case in history. Important changes have taken place over the last thirty years or so in the historiography of the First World War, and research now focuses more closely on the fallen soldiers and the place that European societies have tried to give them. Through pioneering studies on war memorials,[3] war cemeteries, new funerary rites and negotiations over the fate of bodies by states, armies and families, this new history of war has illustrated a history of mourning in the context of the mass deaths of soldiers.[4] Other studies have discussed the presence of corpses in towns on the front line – towns with infirmaries where the wounded had become a part of the social fabric and often the dead as well.[5] In such a vigorous historiography of the European war (the international dimension of the First World War is often neglected in this context), bodies are seen as wounded, broken and reconstructed.

The study of French soldiers with facial injuries was greatly influential in this new relationship with the body; however, these corpses were still not seen as independent social agents.[6] In more general terms, the history of military and wartime medicine has undergone changes due to extensive research on the *body*, in which is seen a field of social forces and representations.

Interestingly, such studies have not yet addressed the Second World War, which had a much higher percentage of civilian deaths. It would appear that research into the Holocaust has avoided paying much attention to the millions of dead bodies that resulted.[7] Conversely, the limited research on the place of the corpse in mass violence and wars has had little impact on the historical analysis of genocide. There again, the body is only briefly addressed, often in discussions on methods of killing. The Holocaust is almost an exception, with detailed, but limited, research on gas chambers, crematoria and, more recently, the organization and techniques used by the mobile death squads in eastern Europe, the *Einsatzgruppen*.[8] Historical research could gain much, however, by considering mass corpses and by studying accounts and sources in order to define the sequence of events that led to the specific treatment of the body at the time of massacre and after. A description of the search and identification processes for corpses could thus contribute to social history, cultural history and the history of medicine. A historiographical approach would demonstrate the administrative structures involved in the treatment of corpses en masse, as well as the structures of power and reappropriation in a context in which the bodies are seen as objects that were subject to ancient or modern techniques originating from other conflicts, from local traditions or even those newly developed. It therefore seems clear that historical research on the memory of mass killings and genocides – research that has increased over the last few decades – would gain much by shifting its focus from monuments and representations (particularly in cultural studies) to the actual sites of the massacres and mass graves. An approach based on individual biographies or cohorts (social sub-groups or groups defined by age) could be used here by historians. A biographical approach from the point of view of the persecutors or the victims or even from the point of view of those responsible for the exhumations and memorials is also a method that a historian could use. Furthermore, specific attention to the chronology and the sequencing of events would be beneficial for studies of corpses in mass violence and genocides.

In order to illustrate the possibilities outlined above for the development of a history of social and political practices related to corpses en masse, I shall discuss the work of the French search mission in Germany, a body that was active from 1946 to 1958 and that was under the charge of the Ministry of War Veterans, Deportees and War Victims.[9] To illustrate the potential of research into the role of the body in – and after – situations of mass violence and genocide, we address two specific aspects: first, the diplomatic dimension of the negotiations that led to the French search mission being given authorization to work on German soil; and second, in greater detail, the use of physical anthropology and forensics in identifying the bodies of French deportees buried in individual and mass graves.

Negotiating diplomatic status

For over ten years the French search mission devoted considerable resources and major financial investments to strengthening its forensics techniques, earthmoving equipment and identification capacity; however, it also needed the support and commitment of diplomats, deportee organizations and the families of those missing. During this time in Germany, a group of French civil servants systematically searched the concentration camps in the Reich and exhumed tens of thousands of corpses and skeletons in order to try to identify French deportees (or rather, deportees from France). Other countries, such as Belgium, Italy and Denmark, organized similar search missions.[10] It is worth noting, however, that, to our knowledge, no mention has been made of the French mission in any of the many books or papers on the subject of the memory of the Holocaust or the consequences of deportation from France. This historiographic silence is interesting in itself, and perhaps implies a certain disembodiment in the accounts of the concentration camps, which tend to focus on the stories of the survivors and to neglect the material aspects of the political treatment of the dead.[11]

Current portrayals of deportation, whether they address racial deportees or resistance fighters, render the body abstract and simply depict the fires in the crematoria of the concentration camps and death camps. Of course, the concentration camp system and the Nazi genocidal system (which it is worth making a distinction between) both required crematoria to be built on a large scale, the most famous of which were those at Birkenau (Auschwitz II).[12]

Some of the deportees' bodies were not incinerated, however, particularly in the final months of the war, due to the increase in the number of deaths and the absence of fuel (wood or coal) for the incinerators. The bodies were then buried in mass graves, either near to the camp or *kommando*,[13] or in the municipal cemeteries or Jewish cemeteries in the neighbouring villages.[14] The prisoners who survived until the concentration camp system was dismantled were then taken on forced 'death marches', in which they were evacuated by foot along the roads of the Reich. Those who fell were shot dead by the SS, and a large number of them died of exhaustion. Their bodies were abandoned on the roadsides or buried quickly and anonymously by local communities.[15]

The liberation of the concentration camps and the occupation of Germany were followed by major search operations for survivors, and estimations of the number of foreigners who had died in the Reich. On 10 December 1945, General Koenig passed an ordinance in the French zone of occupation obliging German municipalities to draw up a list of all the deceased citizens of the allied nations, providing all available details of their names, nationalities and the circumstances of their deaths. Similar statutes were passed in the British and American zones.[16] In the French zone, by the summer of 1946, out of a total of 5,200 communes, 5,090 had provided documents, including 3,959 legal records, 4,600 death certificates and details of 3,982 graves that had been identified. Similar figures were produced in the British and American zones.

The French search mission was under the charge of the Civil Tracing Service for Deportees at the Ministry of Veterans' Affairs. This service was charged with establishing the identities of the survivors and the dead, producing various lists and collating information. From October 1946, changes were made and it was decided that the bodies of French deportees found in the Reich (including those in the Soviet zone of occupation) could be brought back to France, to be buried in the cemetery of the families' choice.[17] Discussions were largely concerned with the material conditions of repatriation (it was difficult to provide real coffins for all the bodies; however, large numbers of shrouds were available as well as sixteen trucks and ten cars), and the bodies that were identified were all brought to Strasbourg before being sent to different towns in France. Deportee associations were already very active at the time and followed the operations closely. They protested regularly at the Ministry; they particularly wanted the families who desired it to be able to be present during the exhumations, but the civil servants tried to avoid this because of the emotion that the exhumations incited, as the bodies were usually found in mass graves. Repatriation took place only on the specific request of the family of the deceased.[18] When the body of a French deportee was identified and no request had been made by the family for repatriation, it was inhumed at a French burial section of the camp site. These sections had been designed according to a military model, and the diplomats in charge of them often had to fight to prevent changes being made to the sites so that their 'French character' could be preserved. A certain 'extraterritoriality' was – and still is today – symbolized by this strict delimitation of the French section and the presence of the French flag.

Towards the end of 1947, the civil servants working for the search mission in Germany lost their military status. With the creation of the Anglo-American bizone, followed by the trizone and finally the Federal Republic, the mission's activities were regrouped into one location, initially Bad Elms and later Bad Neuenahr. The negotiations on the self-government agreement for the Federal Republic of Germany forced it to rethink and to give the French search mission an official status, which led to the signing of the diplomatic Franco-German agreement on 23 October 1954.[19] The negotiations were not concluded for many years, however, and as long as the German state was considered non-existent as a result of the collapse of the Reich in April and May 1945 (as there was no longer a legitimate government) the occupying forces were sovereign in the conquered territory within the limits of the international treaties,[20] particularly the Hague Conventions, and had the right to exhume. Negotiations over access to the sites of the assassinations were in fact held between the Allies, in which the French search mission needed to gain the right to work in the Soviet, British and American zones.

The creation of the Federal Republic of Germany on 23 May 1949 marked a change in legal approach: the French mission, which had up to then an undefined interim status, now found itself in a territory that was regaining a part of its sovereignty. However, the Federal Republic was still under the Occupation Statute, which was to be renegotiated, and the possibility of a peace agreement being reached was becoming rapidly less likely with the definitive partition of Germany. The negotiation of the country's sovereignty (in German, the 'transition treaty') continued up until October 1954. In view of the signing of the treaty, the French authorities brought the question of the small search mission to the negotiating table, fearing that its activity would be stopped for legal reasons.

On 3 September 1953, André François-Poncet, the High Commissioner in Bonn, wrote to the Ministry of War Veterans and War Victims in Paris, more precisely to the Office of War Graves in the Department of Civil Status, to suggest that negotiations be opened up with the Germans in order to determine the definitive status of the search mission.[21] The Ministry of War Veterans was reluctant to open negotiations, but the French Ministry of Foreign Affairs insisted. The Auswärtiges Amt – its German counterpart – had already made contact with the embassy to request that discussions were opened regarding German war graves in France. The Germans considered these negotiations to be a reciprocal act, however, and this created difficulties: 'We must avoid considering in terms of reciprocity a matter that is only a problem for us because of the atrocities carried out by the Germans. It is their duty not to make matters worse through any more or less voluntary negligence in preserving the memory of the deceased', wrote Jean Sauvagnargues, the Director of the European desk at the Ministry of Foreign Affairs, on 1 December 1953.[22] While the Ministry of Foreign Affairs wanted to negotiate, however, the Department of Civil Status at the Ministry of War Veterans was very distrustful of the Germans, as the conservation of the concentration camps and *kommandos* (for memorial purposes), for example, had encountered a number of problems.[23] The local German authorities were embarking on work during this reconstruction period that threatened the integrity of the concentration camps and mass graves. This was an observation that was often made by delegations of survivors or families of the deceased when they visited. The problem was that, up until then, it was the Treaty of Versailles that had been applied in terms of the maintenance of war graves; however, the graves of the deportees were not – or not yet – considered such, and negotiations were aimed at having this redefinition accepted by the Germans. However, the legal positioning of National Socialism meant that the German diplomats considered the deportees as non-regular combatants. According to the Treaty of Versailles, each country should cover the costs of the maintenance of enemy graves on their own territory. France thus spent 82 million francs regrouping and maintaining German graves, but the costs of identifying and regrouping the deportees' bodies in Germany had up until then been covered by France. The search mission remained French but now that it was under the authority of the embassy in Bonn it obtained diplomatic status and the searches received a budgetary allocation from the German federal state.

Negotiations were concluded at the end of May 1954. The Germans had accepted almost all of the French stipulations and two draft conventions had been drawn up, one on 'the consequences of deportation' and the other on German war graves in France.[24] The conventions were to be signed in June 1954. The European desk of the Ministry of Foreign Affairs was delighted with this, as these agreements were likely to ease Franco-German relations: safeguarding the integrity of the concentration camps and the question of German graves in France had created tension on both sides of the Rhine. Germany had also initiated negotiations on the question of graves with a dozen other countries, including Egypt.

Once the text of the convention on the consequences of deportation had been drawn up, the contents of the annexes still needed to be negotiated. They were to address three points: the sum to be paid by the Federal Republic of Germany; the list of exhumations still to be carried out (4,000 were planned); and the list of the 'main sites' of deportation and the erection or maintenance of monuments. The delegations met in Bonn at the Ministry of Foreign Affairs on 10 June 1954. Discussions were tense, but the embassy reported to Paris that the Germans were acting with goodwill.[25]

The agreement was finally signed in Paris by Chancellor Konrad Adenauer on 23 October 1954,[26] and by the Chancellor and Pierre Mendès-France (who at the time was both President of the Cabinet and Minister of Foreign Affairs) during the Franco-German meetings that followed the Nine-Power Conference in Paris on the western military alliance. That day also, the four occupying forces signed an agreement resolving the main problems in Germany (the occupation troops were to remain, but the country was to be granted its full independence), and the Federal Republic of Germany signed a treaty allowing it to join NATO, as well as a convention on cultural exchanges between Germany and France, allowing for student and university trips and the support of language learning.

The French mission's work extended to the whole of the German Federal Republic and, without any particular difficulties, to the German Democratic Republic as well. The Soviet authorities in East Berlin were very helpful in this up until the uprising on 17 June 1953. From this date onwards, exhumations were no longer authorized in the German Democratic Republic.[27] To our knowledge, the search mission did not work outside of these areas, and therefore not in Poland, where Auschwitz and its many *kommandos* were located, and where the death marches involving the highest number of deportees had taken place.

Identifying bodies

How were the exhumations carried out? Initially, documents and survivors' accounts were compiled and compared, and a list of sites to be searched was submitted to the local German authorities. Earth-moving equipment was then transported to the sites (the labourers themselves were German), and sometimes tents were set up to shelter the tables on which the remains were spread. The skeletons were first reassembled at the site itself, and the remains were then transported by truck to the mission's headquarters. The cars used by the French civil servants had diplomatic licence plates (we do not know whether this was also the case for the trucks). At the headquarters the skeletons were photographed and studied in more detail. Up to 1,500 skeletons were stored in the mission's basements. The bodies that were identified as not being 'French' were then either passed on to other search missions (the missions sometimes exchanged remains) or reburied in the same place. From the mass of remains exhumed, relatively few bodies were repatriated. The people in charge of exhuming the bodies were sometimes simply looking for just one body that had been buried at the side of the road after a death march, or at other times opened up enormous mass graves such as that at Vaihingen, which had been a 'hospital' camp for the *kommandos* of the Neckar valley and a terrible death camp for sick deportees. 'In Vaihingen itself, where we identified 270 French bodies, 29 Dutch, 14 Belgian, 13 Norwegian and 18 Italian, the systematic opening of graves began in March 1954', stated an official report by the search mission in April 1955. 'Operations came to an end in September, at which time 1,488 bodies had been exhumed from a total of thirteen graves. The large number of corpses that the majority of the graves contained (one of them had up to 231 bodies) was not an obstacle to identification.'[28] The grave that was opened at Allach, near Dachau, revealed thousands of bodies as well. The search mission handled almost 10,000 corpses there. At Bergen-Belsen, which was the last stage of this major mission, they expected to exhume at least 12,000 bodies. However, at the last minute the exhumations were halted because of protests by the camp's Jewish survivors, who considered the mission's work a desacralization of Jewish graves.[29] These were the most significant protests, but other conflicts had also previously occurred, such as at Donauwörth, where the inhabitants of the nearest village had made complaints that the French civil servants were disturbing the dead. On a few occasions, such as at Ratisbonne in 1960, work took place in the town's cemetery, where the dead deportees from the local *kommando* had been buried in a communal grave.

In order to be able to identify the thousands of dead, the search mission had to use forensics. In October 1953, a delegation of some of the most important French anthropologists and forensic scientists carried out an inspection at one of the exhumation sites. Doctors Vallois, Piédelièvre, Mallet and Garlopeau went to Kochendorf, in the Neckar valley.[30] At the time, René Piédelièvre was the director of the Paris Forensics Institute[31] (l'Institut médico-légal de Paris) and Henri-Victor Vallois was a professor of physical anthropology at the Musée de l'Homme in Paris.[32] As no archives had been found for the *kommando* at Kochendorf, the bodies were identified solely using forms that had been completed by the families. They included an identity photograph of the deportee, a detailed description (height, weight, etc.), details of any distinctive features (past fractures, for example) and dental treatments, filled in by the deceased's former dentist.[33] The doctors reported that at Kochendorf the ground was first surveyed in great detail in order to accurately mark out the limits of the grave. Siliceous clay had not yet entered into the bone structures and so the remains were well preserved. The German technicians then used archaeological methods to remove the earth with a brush so that it slowly revealed the bones. 'The labourers generally begin at the extremities of the bodies with the phalanges, metacarpals, then carpals for the hands, and the phalanges, metatarsals, then tarsals for the feet' wrote the inspectors.[34]

Each skeleton had to be reassembled in order to determine the history of each body and age at the time of death. Specialist German doctors, whose names were not specified, were in charge of this job.[35] Each skull and jaw was photographed using a special camera, as well as 'any bones that had distinctive lesions, past fractures or acquired bone lesions'.[36] If any doubt remained in identifying a particular body, further information was requested from the deportee's likely family. If the body had not been specifically requested, the remains were collected in a plastic bag, which was then placed in a small individual coffin in order to allow for later identification if a subsequent request was received from the family.

The mission's forensic experts provided some feedback in order to improve the procedures. In particular, they suggested that photographs be taken during the course of the exhumations and that any hairs that were found should be analysed. They also asked that skull measurements be taken more systematically and that X-rays be used.

In their report, the four doctors tried to connect the mission's forensic work (looking for bodies) with the traditional work of French forensic scientists; surely the sheer number of bodies studied should allow for certain hypotheses and work methods to be approved or rejected? This was the case for the determination of age and sex. 'The methods used on thousands of skeletons have shown that skeletons usually evolve with age. We believe that this was not very widely known up until now, and that outside of all pathological evolution, an ageing of the bone structure can also be identified' they wrote.[37] They concluded by saying that the archaeological methods used for the exhumations in Germany had never been used in France and that they recommended 'importing' it. On this occasion they recommended that German methods be adopted in France and also that French methods be adopted in Germany.

The search mission thus used traditional forensic identification techniques, their only 'originality' being the extent of their work, which covered thousands of bodies. The German forensic scientist whose work was observed at Kochendorf, for example, was responsible for over 3,500 corpses. In 1957, the mission had exhumed and examined around 50,000 bodies, 7,000 of which had been identified as French (or deportees from France); 4,000 of these 7,000 bodies were repatriated back to France and the others were buried in the French section of the camps. The statistics provided by the mission indicated a high percentage of identification: in Binau, 91 per cent of the French deportees who were searched for were identified; in Haslach 81 per cent; and in Vaihingen 77 per cent.

The search mission demonstrated a clear continuity of military practices in the treatment of the bodies. Following the First World War, in order to respond to the high numbers of requests by families and war veterans' associations, a law was passed to allow the bodies buried in the battlefields to be exhumed. This vast undertaking in Germany was thus in accordance with the law of 31 July 1920 which ordained that the bodies of fallen soldiers be repatriated to family cemeteries at the expense of the state. During the period in question, the mission principally sought to identify the bodies of political deportees and resistance fighters, but in application of the strict post-war memorial policy, which refused any distinctions between political and racial deportees (with the exception of pensions, which were higher for political deportees), the families of the Jewish deportees were also able to benefit from the law. Research was nonetheless limited to the new borders of the two Germanys following the Potsdam conference, and the six Nazi death camps installed in Poland remained outside the mission's jurisdiction. Two aspects of the mission's work are of special interest here: first, the sorting of bodies represented a huge undertaking; and second, only the bodies of French deportees (even if it was a question of Jews or foreign resistance fighters) were searched for and were subject to identification procedures. The 'inappropriate' bodies – those of other deportees – did not interest the mission. Furthermore, one of its main concerns was to ensure that it did not repatriate 'inappropriate' French bodies, in other words those of voluntary workers in Germany and above all collaborators who took refuge in the Reich at the end of the war and died there. As their remains were buried in Frohnau cemetery in Berlin, the people in charge of the digs in the cemetery were particularly careful to ensure that the bodies of the deportees were not confused with or, worse still, mixed up with those of people considered traitors to the nation.

The search mission was dismantled slowly from 1956 onwards. The last exhumations were to take place in Bergen-Belsen and were planned to be on a massive scale, considering the specific history of the camp (over 20,000 inmates had died there in the weeks before and after the liberation). Even before they started, the exhumations were contested by the central organization of Jews in Germany and by the body of Bergen-Belsen survivors. It provoked a long controversy between the French authorities and the French deportees' organizations on one side, and the German government and Jewish organizations from all over the world on the other. Exhumations in Bergen-Belsen consequently never took place, following a decision from an international arbitration commission.[38]

The work of the search mission came to an end because the demands for exhumations ceased to be lodged and the endeavour was considered as finished by the French Ministry of War Veterans and the deportees' organizations.

The French search mission first worked under the framework of a military occupation, and this role remained unchanged till it was dismantled. But in the twelve years of its existence, French–German relations tremendously evolved. From arch-enemies, the two nations started a slow but very significant redefinition of their relationship, towards friendship, reconciliation and then a strong alliance, an alliance formally established in Paris in January 1963. However, the search mission did not play a significant role in this coming to terms with centuries of war and conflict. It was seen by the French only as a precondition for further negotiations and this was constantly repeated by diplomats. But the very activities of the mission – the exhumations – were not given much publicity beyond the circles of deportees and their families. The reconciliation process was built far more on silence over deportation and the Holocaust, or at least on a narrative of common resistance to National Socialism that had taken place in the concentration camps.

The search mission was an undertaking that involved re-nationalizing corpses, but it did not have solely nationalistic aims: it also allowed for the reprivatization of the bodies. The families who were waiting for them to be returned were aware of what was at stake. Thus the Duchess of Ayen, whose husband, Jean de Noailles d'Ayen, had been deported to Germany and died in Bergen-Belsen on 13 April 1945, wrote on the subject of the search mission to Maurice Couve de Murville, who had just been appointed Minister of Foreign Affairs. She said the mission's work was 'admirably conducted and carried out and had already proven its moral efficiency (without mentioning its scientific expertise), with the final aim being – far from desecrating the remains – to return those who died for their country to the grave that they deserved, a grave that would preserve their identity with the memory of their sacrifice … all things that the Nazi camps had wanted to abolish'.[39]

Notes

1 The text of this chapter was translated from the author's French by Cadenza Academic Translations.
2 See the numerous studies on the Middle Ages and modern times, such as J. Delumeau, *Une histoire du paradis* (Paris: Fayard, 1992); P. Ariès, *L'Homme devant la mort* (Paris: Le Seuil, 1977); P. Ariès, *Essais sur l'histoire de la mort en Occident: du Moyen-Âge à nos jours* (Paris: Le Seuil, 1975).
3 See for example A. Prost, 'Les monuments aux morts. Cultes républicains? Culte civique? Culte patriotique?', in P. Nora (ed.), *Les Lieux de mémoire* (Paris: Gallimard, Quarto, 1997), vol. 1, pp. 199–223.
4 There is a wealth of literature on the subject, for example J.-J. Becker, 'L'évolution de l'historiographie de la Première Guerre mondiale', *Revue Historique des Armées*, 242 (2006) (special issue, *1916, les grandes batailles et la fin de la guerre européenne*), pp. 4–15; A. Prost & J. Winter, *The Great War in History: Debates and Controversies, 1914 to the Present* (Cambridge: Cambridge University Press, 2005).
5 See in particular the work of Roger Chickering on the town of Freiburg/Breisgau, in the Grand Duchy of Baden (Germany): R. Chickering, *The Great War and Urban Life in Germany: Freiburg, 1914–1918* (Cambridge: Cambridge University Press, 2007).

6 S. Delaporte, *Les Gueules cassées: les blessés de la face de la Grande Guerre* (Paris: Editions Noêsis, 1996); A. Carden-Coyne, *Reconstructing the Body: Classicism, Modernism, and the First World War* (Oxford: Oxford University Press, 2009).
7 On the subject of mourning rituals in France during the Second World War, see nonetheless: D. Voldman & L. Capdevila, *Nos morts: les sociétés occidentales face aux tués de la guerre, XIXe–XXe siècles* (Paris: Payot, 2002).
8 H. Krausnick, *Hitlers Einsatzgruppen: die Truppe des Weltanschauungskrieges, 1938–1942* (Frankfurt am Main: Fischer, 1985); H. C. Earl, *The Nuremberg SS-Einsatzgruppen Trial, 1945–1958* (Cambridge: Cambridge University Press, 2009).
9 The mission's research activities have been very briefly discussed in J.-M. Dreyfus, 'Conflits de mémoires autour du cimetière de Bergen-Belsen', *Vingtième Siècle: Revue d'Histoire*, 90 (2006), pp. 73–87; that article was reprinted in M.-B. Vincent (ed.), *La Dénazification* (Paris: Perrin, 2008), pp. 235–57.
10 For more on the Danish search mission, see S. A. Birkeland, *I krigens kølvand* (Copenhagen: Gyldendal, 2009).
11 The research for this chapter was mainly carried out using the archives at the French Ministry of Foreign Affairs. The files concerning the search mission were from a range of sources from different French diplomatic posts in the Federal Republic of Germany. I completed my research by reading a few files from the Auswärtiges Amt, the German Ministry of Foreign Affairs, particularly those relating to the Franco-German Convention on 'the consequences of deportation' in 1954. I also used an inspection report by French forensic scientists, published in the *Bulletin de l'Académie de Médecine* (1955, no. 16).
12 The most comprehensive study of the crematoria of Auschwitz is the remarkable book by Robert Jan van Pelt which discusses the case for the defence in the Irving trial: R. J. van Pelt, *The Case for Auschwitz: Evidence from the Irving Trial* (Bloomington: Indiana University Press, 2002).
13 A *kommando* was, in the vocabulary of concentration camps, a 'sub-camp' that was an offspring of a larger camp.
14 See, for example, the case of Echterdingen, a *kommando* of Struthof-Natzwiller, who was located on the German bank of the Rhine. J.-M. Dreyfus, 'Echterdingen', in G. Megargee (ed.), *The United States Holocaust Memorial Museum Encyclopedia of Camps and Ghettos, 1933–1945* (Bloomington: Indiana University Press, 2009), vol. 1, pp. 1027–8, at p. 1027. The bodies were buried in the forest near the *kommando*.
15 On the death marches, see the book by Daniel Blatman, *Les Marches de la mort: la dernière* étape *du génocide nazi, été 1944–printemps 1945* (Paris: Fayard, 2009); and also the beautiful book by Robert Antelme, *L'Espèce humaine* (Paris: Gallimard, 1999 – original edition 1957), p. 220.
16 For the British zone, the decree dates to 29 January 1946.

17 See the preparation meetings for the first repatriations in Archives nationales, Paris, F9 3843.
18 The letters that were sent together with the administrative forms were evidently very emotional and moving as they retraced the events in the life of a young resistance fighter or member of a Jewish family in a very concise manner.
19 Franco-German Convention on 'the consequences of deportation', signed by Pierre Mendès-France and Konrad Adenauer on 23 October 1954 in Paris.
20 There is insufficient research on the status of corpses (and exhumations) in international law.
21 Centre des archives diplomatiques de Nantes (henceforth CADN), Embassy of Bonn, no. 20, Dispatch by the Ministry of Foreign Affairs, European Department – Central Europe Division at the embassy of Bad Godesberg, regarding the problems of maintenance of civil and military war graves after the contractual agreements came into force on 1 December 1953.
22 Jean Sauvagnargues, 1915–2002. A former student at the École Normale Supérieure, and member of the Foreign Office, Sauvagnargues joined France Libre in 1943. He was a member of Général de Gaulle's cabinet during the Liberation, Director of German and Austrian Affairs at the Ministry of Foreign Affairs, Minister of Foreign Affairs in 1955 during Antoine Pinay's second government, then ambassador in Ethiopia and Tunisia. He was ambassador in Bonn from 1970 to 1974, and then Minister of Foreign Affairs for Valéry Giscard d'Estaing's first government.
23 CADN, Embassy of Bonn, no. 20, Letter from the Ministry of War Veterans and War Victims, Office of War Graves, at the Ministry of Foreign Affairs, Central Europe Division, 22 October 1953. See also the minutes of the preparatory meeting in Bonn, Politisches Archiv des Auswärtigen Amtes (PAAA; Political Archives of the Ministry of Foreign Affairs), Berlin, B86 1372, Aktenvermerk, Betr. Ausländische Kriegggräber in Deutschland, Exhumierung von ausländischen Kriegstoten, 21 August 1953, meeting of 29 October 1953.
24 CADN, Embassy of Bonn, no. 20, Letter from the Ministry of Foreign Affairs, Central Europe Division, Jean Sauvagnargues to High Commissioner, ambassador, 31 May 1954.
25 CADN, Embassy of Bonn, no. 20, Dispatch no. 1243 concerning Franco-German negotiations on some of the problems resulting from deportation and regarding the maintenance of German military graves in France, 10 June 1954. It should be noted that the correspondence exchanged between Paris and Bonn on the subject of the agreement was copied from this date onwards to the Minister's Office, which remained Georges Bidault's office for two more days. On 14 June, Pierre Mendès-France, who had become President of the Council, took over the Ministry of Foreign Affairs.
26 In his memoirs, Adenauer provides not more than a list of treaties and agreements signed on that day, including the Convention on 'the

The French search mission for corpses 143

consequences of deportation': K. Adenauer, *Erinerungen 1953–1955* (Stuttgart: Deutsche Verlags-Anstalt, 1966), p. 382.
27 See the negotiations on this subject: CADN, Embassy of Bonn, no. 28.
28 CADN, Embassy of Bonn, no. 20, Letter no. 52349, Ministry of War Veterans to the High Commissioner, 26 April 1955, pp. 7–9.
29 On this debate, which lasted for over ten years and which was finally decided by a diplomatic arbitration committee, see Dreyfus, 'Conflits de mémoires'.
30 This mission resulted in a detailed scientific report and a large number of photographs. It was also the subject of a statement to the Academy of Medicine, and the subsequent publication of an article: H. V. Vallois, R. Piédelièvre, P. Mallet & S. Garlopeau, 'Données anthropologiques et médico-légales concernant l'identification des squelettes', *Bulletin de l'Académie Nationale de Médecine*, 119:3 (1955), pp. 67–80.
31 René Piédelièvre wrote a memoir: R. Piédèlievre, *Souvenirs d'un médecin légiste* (Paris: Flammarion, 1966).
32 On Vallois' activity see Y. Coppens, 'Le professeur Henri-Victor Vallois, anthropologue et paléoanthropologue', *Bulletin et Mémoire de la Société d'Anthropologie de Paris*, 9:9–2 (1982), pp. 103–7.
33 I consulted the copies of 254 forms provided for exhumation requests in Bergen-Belsen and I was struck by the scarcity of information. For example, very few of the forms had been completed by dentists.
34 Vallois *et al.*, 'Données anthropologiques', p. 68.
35 Were these doctors trained in forensic medicine under the Nazi regime?
36 Vallois *et al.*, 'Données anthropologiques', p. 68.
37 Ibid., p. 80.
38 See a description of the controversy that was finally closed in 1969 in J.-M. Dreyfus, 'Conflits de mémoires'.
39 Archives at the Ministry of Foreign Affairs, La Courneuve, Minister's Office, Maurice Couve de Murville, no. 296, Letter dated 29 May 1958.

Bibliography

Adenauer, K., *Erinerungen 1953–1955* (Stuttgart: Deutsche Verlags-Anstalt, 1966)
Antelme, R., *L'Espèce humaine* (Paris: Gallimard, 1999 – original edition 1957)
Ariès, P., *Essais sur l'histoire de la mort en Occident: du Moyen-Âge à nos jours* (Paris: Le Seuil, 1975)
Ariès, P., *L'Homme devant la mort* (Paris: Le Seuil, 1977)
Becker, J.-J., 'L'évolution de l'historiographie de la Première Guerre mondiale', *Revue Historique des Armées*, 242 (2006) (special issue, *1916, les grandes batailles et la fin de la guerre européenne*), pp. 4–15
Birkeland, S.A., *I krigens kølvand* (Copenhagen: Gyldendal, 2009)
Blatman, D., *Les Marches de la mort: la dernière étape du génocide nazi, été 1944–printemps 1945* (Paris: Fayard, 2009)

Bulletin de l'Académie de médecine (1955, no. 16)
Carden-Coyne, A., *Reconstructing the Body: Classicism, Modernism, and the First World War* (Oxford: Oxford University Press, 2009)
Chickering, R., *The Great War and Urban Life in Germany: Freiburg, 1914–1918* (Cambridge: Cambridge University Press, 2007)
Coppens, Y., 'Le professeur Henri-Victor Vallois, anthropologue et paléoanthropologue', *Bulletin et Mémoire de la Société d'Anthropologie de Paris*, 9:9–2 (1982), pp. 103–7
Delaporte, S., *Les Gueules cassées: les blessés de la face de la Grande Guerre* (Paris: Editions Noêsis, 1996)
Delumeau, J., *Une histoire du paradis* (Paris: Fayard, 1992)
Dreyfus, J.-M., 'Conflits de mémoires autour du cimetière de Bergen-Belsen', *Vingtième Siècle: Revue d'Histoire*, 90 (2006), pp. 73–87; reprinted in M.-B. Vincent (ed.), *La Dénazification* (Paris: Perrin, 2008), pp. 235–57
Dreyfus, J.-M., 'Echterdingen', in G. Megargee (ed.), *The United States Holocaust Memorial Museum Encyclopedia of Camps and Ghettos, 1933–1945* (Bloomington: Indiana University Press, 2009), vol. 1, pp. 1027–8
Earl, H. C., *The Nuremberg SS-Einsatzgruppen Trial, 1945–1958* (Cambridge: Cambridge University Press, 2009)
Krausnick, H., *Hitlers Einsatzgruppen: die Truppe des Weltanschauungskrieges, 1938–1942* (Frankfurt am Main: Fischer, 1985)
Piédelièvre, R., *Souvenirs d'un médecin légiste* (Paris: Flammarion, 1966)
Prost, A., 'Les monuments aux morts. Cultes républicains? Culte civique? Culte patriotique?', in P. Nora (ed.), *Les Lieux de mémoire* (Paris: Gallimard, Quarto, 1997), vol. 1, pp. 199–223
Prost, A. & J. Winter, *The Great War in History: Debates and Controversies, 1914 to the Present* (Cambridge: Cambridge University Press, 2005)
Vallois, M.-G., J. Piédelièvre, P. Mallet & S. Garlopeau, 'Données anthropologiques et médico-légales concernant l'identification des squelettes', *Bulletin de l'Académie Nationale de Médecine*, 119:3 (1955), pp. 67–80
van Pelt, R. J., *The Case for Auschwitz: Evidence from the Irving Trial* (Bloomington: Indiana University Press, 2002)
Voldman, D. & L. Capdevila, *Nos morts: les sociétés occidentales face aux tués de la guerre, XIXe–XXe siècles* (Paris: Payot, 2002)

Archival sources

Archives at the Ministry of Foreign Affairs, La Courneuve, Minister's Office, Maurice Couve de Murville, no. 296, Letter dated 29 May 1958
Archives nationales, Paris, F9 3843
Centre des archives diplomatiques de Nantes (CADN; Centre for diplomatic archives in Nantes), Embassy of Bonn, no. 20, Dispatch by the Ministry of Foreign Affairs, European Department – Central Europe Division at the embassy of Bad Godesberg, regarding the problems of maintenance of civil and military war graves after the contractual agreements came into force on 1 December 1953

CADN, Embassy of Bonn, no. 20, Dispatch no. 1243 concerning Franco-German negotiations on some of the problems resulting from deportation and regarding the maintenance of German military graves in France, 10 June 1954

CADN, Embassy of Bonn, no. 20, Letter from the Ministry of War Veterans and War Victims, Office of War Graves, at the Ministry of Foreign Affairs, Central Europe Division, 22 October 1953

CADN, Embassy of Bonn, no. 20, Letter from the Ministry of Foreign Affairs, Central Europe Division, Jean Sauvagnargues to High Commissioner, ambassador, 31 May 1954

CADN, Embassy of Bonn, no. 20, Letter no. 52349 from the Ministry of War Veterans to the High Commissioner CADN, 26 April 1955

CADN, Embassy of Bonn, no. 28

Politisches Archiv des Auswärtigen Amtes (PAAA; Political Archives of the Ministry of Foreign Affairs), Berlin, B86 1372, Aktenvermerk, Betr. Ausländische Krieggräber in Deutschland, Exhumierung von ausländischen Kriegstoten, 21 August 1953, meeting of 29 October 1953

7

From bones-as-evidence to tutelary spirits: the status of bodies in the aftermath of the Khmer Rouge genocide

Anne Yvonne Guillou

Introduction

'What is a body?' The question asked by Stéphane Breton is one that haunts those anthropologists who have to deal with any aspect of the materiality of flesh and of its corruption.[1] On the one hand there is its materiality, through which the marks of mass violence such as that of the Khmer Rouge genocide can be read,[2] while on the other there is its corruption, the slow process accompanying the change in the religious status of the corpse as it moves towards different forms of existence, and all the rituals relating to this change.[3] While these definitions of the body are well established within the field of anthropology, the student of genocide must also take into account an additional dimension, namely that of the specific political and legal issues raised by mass violence.

I describe in this chapter the ways in which, during my research, I have come to consider corpses of mass violence in Cambodia, and how the question of observation schedules and temporality seems to me to be fundamental to our understanding of post-genocide Cambodian society, and in particular rural Khmer society, which has been largely neglected since ethnological studies slowly started again in the 1990s.

From the suffering body to scars on the landscape: an ethnography of the traces of the genocide

When, in 2007, I began a programme of ethnographic research into the traces of the Khmer Rouge genocide in a village in western Cambodia, the 'body' that I imagined I would be studying would be of the sort conceptualized by medical anthropology. Healthy body, sick body, dying body: from this perspective, the body is where all disorders are visible, and where the potential reforging of the links between the individual, society and the universe is promised. It is also the site upon which the traces of structural violence and the relations of social domination are inscribed. During my previous research, I had begun to realize that certain forms of illness were thought of as being linked to the suffering endured under the revolutionary regime of the Party of Democratic Kampuchea.[4] A particular example is the syndrome of *bak komlang*, permanently 'broken strength' due to excessively hard labour, leading to a state of apathy and weakness. Through these popular aetiologies, Cambodians have engaged in a sort of spontaneous political anthropology, analysing destructive events through their most visibly corporeal consequences.[5]

I had thus embarked upon the project of 'reading' the genocide through the traces left on bodies and psyches, as described by rural Khmers. However, two events, one occurring during a meeting in Paris, the other on a country road in Cambodia, led me to widen my perspective and 'leave the body' of medical anthropology. The first was a remark made to me by Anne-Christine Taylor while I was describing the craters left by American bombs along the length of the border between Cambodia and Vietnam. Why, she asked, was I limiting the scope of my enquiry to the bodily traces of the years of war and genocide, and not linking these to the traces left on the landscape? Her remark came back to me a few months later when I was driving around the Cardamom region, between Lake Tonle Sap and the forested plateau in the west of Cambodia, in search of a village to play host to my new project. The name of one sub-district, *snam preah*, grabbed my attention. *Snam preah* means 'mark of the sacred one' in Khmer, and usually refers to the footprints of the Buddha, whose travels, according to legend, took him through all the Theravada Buddhist societies of South-East Asia. Yet *snam* also denotes bodily scars. Since the Khmer language itself had led me in this direction, I refocused my attention away from the 'body' towards the landscape, and from the landscape onto the 'traces' of many kinds left by the mass destruction of thirty years earlier.

In the village of Kompong Tralach,[6] which I had selected for my study, I began, free of any preconceptions, to study what the villagers saw as being its history, based on its most important sites – all places linked to Buddhism, the monarchy or the cult of the area's tutelary 'spirits'.[7] I had benefited in this respect from a degree of luck in my choice of village. When looking for a village willing to play host to my research, I had begun by selecting a specific area in Pursat province which possessed the macro-sociological characteristics I sought.[8] For I wanted to carry out my research in a region representative of Cambodia in terms of its inhabitants' way of life (subsistence rice farming in the rainy season; location away from the Vietnamese, Thai and Laotian borders and the specific cultural issues these raise; well established history of stable settlement, away from zones of large-scale forest clearance which also raises specific questions). It was also important that the zone in question should have suffered disproportionately under Pol Pot's regime. As the historian David Chandler has noted:

> the worst conditions of all were probably in dambon [Khmer Rouge district] 2 and 6 in Pursat,[9] where new people were made to carve villages out of malarial forest. In these zones, deaths from starvation, disease and overwork were frequent, while CPK [Communist Party of Kampuchea] cadre[s] suffered from regional purges in 1976 and 1978. They were replaced, here and in the northwest, by cadres brought in from the Southwestern Zone, the area controlled by Ta Mok, who earned a fearful personal reputation in the DK [Democratic Kampuchea] era and after.[10]

Furthermore, following the rebellion by party cadres in the eastern zone in 1978, thousands of people were deported from Svay Rieng and Prey Veng to Pursat, where they were massacred. Many of them wore traditional blue Khmer scarves (*krama*), and some villagers have told me of the fear and pity that they felt on seeing these deportees who were so clearly marked out as different.[11]

I had travelled around the region in the company of a Cambodian archaeologist friend who had introduced me to the head of the Department of Culture for Pursat, with a view to him helping me with my research. He took me to see the sanctuary of a powerful local tutelary spirit, Grandfather Khleang Mueng, the upkeep of which was his responsibility. According to the royal chronicles and stories told locally, Khleang Mueng was a sixteenth-century military leader who, faced with the Siamese armies, supposedly committed suicide in order to pass into the kingdom of the dead and raise an army of ghosts able to put the enemy to flight. As a national hero, he is venerated not only by local villagers but also by passing travellers and the kingdom's ruling classes. The space of the village, then, is punctuated and structured by a series of sites (altars, monasteries, places with special names) which are all linked to Khleang Mueng's sanctuary and his story. In the context of my 'anthropology of traces', I have thus observed the marks of two superimposed pasts: the war between the Siamese and the Khmer in the sixteenth century, and the Khmer Rouge regime in the twentieth century, which both left behind traces of blood and tears in (virtually) the same places. These traces can be read in built structures, the discourse and stories surrounding them, and the social practices linked to them.

Much as an archaeologist would, I observed how these sites had come through the intervening time, in particular the years of the American war and the Khmer Rouge regime. For instance, a canal dug using forced labour under the Democratic Kampuchean regime 'violently' cuts through the sanctuary of Grandfather Khleang Mueng, a monumental statue of the Buddha has been hacked away at with pickaxes, great trees possessing a powerful aura have been felled. These mutilations, this violence that the villagers helped me to read in the landscape and in these important sites, are metaphors for the violence inflicted upon individuals, a violence which is more difficult to speak about not only because of the way in which Khmer society deals with the expression of painful emotion, but also because of its vision of the relationship between the living and the dead.[12] The language of places thus constituted a basis for discussions with the people of the village. It allowed me to bring out certain spatio-temporal categories generally present in Khmer thought, and understand where, within this general intellectual framework, the brutal split constituted by the Khmer Rouge regime was situated. For among these scars on the landscape were mass graves left by the Pol Potists, with their discreet presence unnoticed by the casual traveller: burial pits scattered across the coutryside, punctuating the rice paddies, the stretches of bush grazed by water buffalo, and the land surrounding pagodas.

The intrusion of corpses into public space at a village and national level

Hundreds of dead at the village level, and hundreds of thousands at the national level, have invaded Cambodians' physical and mental space, the product of the stated wish of the Pol Pot regime to abolish the frontier between the living and the dead.[13] The blurring of these distinctions may be placed in the more general context of Khmer Rouge agrarian totalitarian ideology, which saw rice production, the march of Cambodian history and individual destinies as a single unified whole. This can be seen, for example, in the slogans chanted during this period, such as 'die on the building site' (describing the most glorious death possible) or 'keeping you alive brings us nothing, eliminating you costs us nothing', which was a threat repeated over and over by Khmer Rouge guards. According to the socio-political groups in question,[14] and according to the geostrategic developments that have occurred since the fall of the regime in 1979, different temporal perspectives coexist, turning the Khmer Rouge genocide into a question with constantly shifting boundaries in which bodies, which are ceaselessly redefined and 'renovated', occupy a central position. Human remains have thus been variously defined and treated as corpses, dead people, ghosts, ancestors, bones-as-evidence and bones-as-memorials. They have subsequently been subjected to a range of different physical, ritual, discursive and museographic treatments which have transformed and arranged them, made them 'speak' or 'keep silent'. One gets a sense of the multiplicity of these definitions and their ramifications when one spends time living in Cambodian villages, all the while listening out for the muffled echoes coming from Phnom Penh, where the Khmer Rouge Tribunal has been working since 2007, and keeping an eye on related reports in the international media.

In late 1978, Vietnamese tanks pushed back their erstwhile Khmer Rouge allies in order to put an end to escalating cross-border attacks. The surviving Cambodians, haggard and exhausted, left their collective farms and took to the roads first in search of food, then to look for their missing loved ones or their family homes. In the ensuing months, many of them would live surrounded by corpses: corpses left scattered across the fields following hastily executed massacres of the civilian population during the retreat of Khmer Rouge fighters and cadres towards the Thai border; corpses piled up outside infirmaries and political prisons; isolated corpses of individuals who had collapsed from exhaustion; the remains of 'traitors' executed by overly zealous young soldiers. The Democratic Kampuchean regime left 1.7 million dead out of a total of 7 million inhabitants, some of whom were identified and buried, most of whom were left where they lay. People have described to me the indifference they felt faced with this spectacle, used as they were to living and sleeping amid these corpses, so racked by hunger that their emotions were utterly numbed. Once the foul smell of putrefaction had subsided, the vast numbers of skulls and bones became a familiar sight for children in these areas, and these human remains continue to resurface in a macabre form of archaeology whenever a well or a ditch is dug. Glowing lights and apparitions, sometimes associated with malevolent 'spirits' known as *priey* which inhabit certain trees, were frequent in the 1980s, then became more intermittent.

As the survivors set about rebuilding their lives, whether in their own former dwellings or in those left vacant by the disappearance of their owners, they would all carry out certain rudimentary rites to allow them to cohabit with the unknown dead who surrounded them: bones would be stacked beneath large trees, cremations would be carried out. At a time when people still had no news of their own family members sent to other areas of the country, these bodies were, in this period, simply corpses from which they sought to distance themselves physically in order to help rekindle their desire to live. This comes across in countless remarks made regarding the insistence with which people spoke of clearing up and cultivating sites of massacres (often in areas of forest or bush), in an effort to transform the raw/wild/forested/uncontrolled into something cooked/domesticated/cultivated/ritualized, in line with Lévi-Straussian symbolic oppositions, which play a deep structuring role in the mental universe of the Khmer.

Bones-as-evidence: ossuaries and memorials from the 1980s to the 2000s

It was on the initiative of the new government put in place under effective Vietnamese control in 1979 that the first collective treatment of the bodies from the genocide was undertaken, its aim being to turn them into 'bones-as-evidence'. This treatment formed part of the general effort to legitimize the new government in the highly polarized international context of the Cold War and the end of the Vietnam War (1975). The invasion of Cambodia by Vietnam was condemned by the west and by communist China (Democratic Kampuchea's principal backer), which persisted in recognizing only the coalition government in exile, of which the Khmer Rouge formed a part.[15] Within the country, too, Cambodians were unsure about what to make of this foreign military presence and this regime that professed to be communist while proclaiming that Pol Pot had betrayed the revolution. Among the steps taken to convince people of the legitimacy of the country's new rulers were the trial *in absentia* of Pol Pot and Ieng Sary by a revolutionary people's court, the transformation of Tuol Sleng prison (known as S-21) into a museum, the opening to the public of Choeung Ek (a site of mass execution near Phnom Penh), the dispatching of investigators into the provinces in order to estimate the numbers who died and, lastly, the construction of memorials.[16] No fewer than eighty small constructions were thus built throughout the country over the 1980s with the assistance of local authorities and villagers, who were asked to gather up the bones scattered across the countryside. Remains which had been thrown down wells, a procedure often used to dispose of bodies after executions, were not exhumed.

Until the peace accords signed in 1991, these memorials would form the backbone of the state's memorialization effort, reaffirming, through annual ceremonies, the cruelty of the Khmer Rouge regime embodied in Pol Pot, the legitimacy of the Vietnamese intervention and the reconciliation programme, which sought to pardon defecting Khmer Rouge cadres and prevent revenge attacks by the people – a typical state programme after genocide or civil war. As well as constituting evidence, then, these human remains also functioned, on a symbolic level, as the foundations upon which the new political order of the People's Republic of Kampuchea would be built. Their significance is clear from the care taken in preparing the bones for the museum at Choeung Ek,[17] and the 'loans' of human remains by sub-district authorities for large-scale regional ceremonies. An even clearer symbol of this new Cambodia built upon the bodies of its children was the immense map of the country made entirely from human skulls which was for many years mounted on a wall of the museum of the genocide at Tuol Sleng prison.

Following the 1991 peace accords, which were signed by all parties, including the Khmer Rouge guerrillas, still known as the Party of Democratic Kampuchea, and the placing of Cambodia under United Nations supervision, any reference to the genocide was not allowed in official documents. The state memorials fell into disrepair. More than fifteen years later, in 2007, at the end of this 'suspended historicity',[18] human remains once again became bones-as-evidence when teams of investigators from the Khmer Rouge Tribunal began recording afresh the sites of massacres, mass graves and political prisons, this work having been started a few years earlier by the Documentation Centre of Cambodia. In parallel with this re-discovery of the country's ossuaries by western agencies, genocide tourism began to develop around the main sites linked to Pol Pot's regime. In Phnom Penh today, one can hear taxi and auto-rickshaw drivers mechanically reciting a litany of sites to tourists, a list of ghastly curiosities to spice up a boat tour on the Mekong river or a visit to the 'silk villages'. In Preah Vihear province, a few metres from the Thai border, Pol Pot's cenotaph and a few other symbolic sites of the Khmer Rouge insurgency in the 1990s are also the object of what is – for the moment at least – a low-key effort by the Tourism Ministry to repackage them as heritage sites.

While the state memorialization project implemented in the 1980s undoubtedly had a strategic aim, this was not its only function. It also allowed the first collective funerary rites to take place, at a time when Buddhism was only just tolerated. The few monks who were allowed by the ruling party to don their habits participated in the ceremonies performed at the memorials and helped transform the anonymous bodies of the genocide into 'spirits of the departed'. With the political liberalization at the beginning of the 1990s and the re-establishment of religious ceremonies, these departed spirits would come to an annual meeting with the living in Buddhist monasteries on the most important date in the Khmer ceremonial calendar, the Festival of the Dead.[19] In relation to these funerary rites, I again followed my chosen methodology for the project by eschewing any framework based on the narrow perspective of genocide, an etic notion which does not correspond to the experiences of the villagers, and instead examined the full range of Buddhist ritual (or textual) procedures for the treatment of the dead – their categorization, their post-mortem trajectory – in order to establish where, specifically or otherwise, the victims of Pol Potism fit into them. It turns out that the treatment of the latter depends not on the specific details of their death, but on their links to the living (whether they have surviving families or remain unidentified[20]) and on the context of the rituals, some of which are rooted in Buddhism (as it is understood and practised in Cambodia across various segments of society, at any rate) and others of which are rooted in what, for our purposes, can be called an ancestor cult.

From earth-bodies to ancestors and tutelary spirits

Among the various categories of victims produced by Democratic Kampuchea is that of the unidentified dead buried in mass graves. From the perspective of Khmer village memorialization, these burial pits are important insofar as they place corpses and landscape on a continuum. For the bodies in these mass graves, now mixed with the earth, absorbed by it, have themselves become earth.[21] This focus on the soil, earth, landscape, all elements which are clearly central to a farming culture, led me down this route of enquiry. During this phase of my research, I deliberately ceased any type of biographical interviewing, and instead concentrated on observing rituals involving the earth and discussing them at length with the people of Kompong Tralach, both religious specialists and ordinary villagers.[22] In such a context, the limits of the biographical interview become very clear.[23] Centred on one person, forcing questions and responses into the mould of concepts of individual suffering, it prevents any collective symbolization and expression of pain.[24]

Today, the way in which people perceive these remains, which emerge from the ground from time to time, during ploughing or the digging of foundations for a house, is complex. On the one hand, they fit into the concept of the earth as being rich in 'treasures' of all kinds.[25] Likewise, the time spent by bodies – of any type – in the ground is considered to enrich the earth, allowing it to 'grow' and prosper.[26] Indeed, one village custom which has often passed unnoticed, or been misinterpreted, consists in performing, usually for people who have died 'normally', a sort of double funeral in which the dead are first buried for several years, after which their remains are exhumed and cremated. I have often heard villagers express an interpretation of this practice in which a certain Buddhist 'conformism' is detectable, insofar as cremation is considered the norm but is often deferred for reasons linked to the cost of the ceremony. A few years after burial, they say, when enough money has been saved, collective funerals shared by several families from the village are organized, during which a cremation is performed. However, my own hypothesis is that, on the contrary, far from being purely contingent on circumstances, the burial of bodies reveals a strong religious dimension. Cambodia's soil is thus made from the bodies of its children who have died throughout its history.

In something of a perversion of this concept, the Khmer Rouge claimed that these bodies served as fertilizer in the fields. And this is precisely what was told to me by one old woman[27] who lived near a pond in which several dozen corpses were found, and which is now used as a reservoir for the rice paddies. 'No one uses this water for cooking because it fills us with disgust, but we do eat fish from this pond.' Then she added, with a dose of peasant humour, 'The fish are nice and plump as well'.

The linking of these bodies to the earth and to specific places contributes to their integration into the category of village tutelary spirits (*neak ta*). Once again, it was by travelling through these ritual sites, in particular the site consecrated to the powerful tutelary spirit Grandfather Khleang Mueng described above, that I was able to draw parallels between the ways in which the villagers perceive certain mass graves and the land's tutelary spirit cults. Khleang Mueng is himself a former human being who died a violent death in the sixteenth century and, like him, other (although not all) tutelary spirits in the region are former human beings who died a cruel death.[28] Their origins vary, having their source both in ancient cults of the power of the soil and in their status as 'ancestors' who cleared the land for the village. This is why Ang Choulean speaks of them quite rightly as 'ancestor[s] blended with the soil'.[29]

There are indeed similarities, at a village level, between the natural abodes of the land's tutelary spirits, such as groves, certain trees, termite hills or other mounds, and certain mass graves. Both are in various ways 'active' and potentially dangerous spaces, where human beings must show respect and caution. For tutelary spirits of the land are rather haughty masters of their territory, jealously guarding the space that they control and protect. Anyone who carelessly trespasses onto the territory of the tutelary spirit without first coming to pay homage to him or her, or who dares to pick fruit without permission, is supposedly punished by illness or, if they give serious offence, death. The relationship established with the tutelary spirit is a relationship of homage from the villagers. An annual ceremony is thus performed at the altars of the more important spirits, at which the local authorities, along with the villagers and monks, are all present. The rest of the time, the relations between the living and the land's tutelary spirits are based on a system of exchange in which humans ask for the help of the *neak ta* in particular circumstances (such as improving a business, make a lover come back, succeeding in an exam) and in return promise to present the spirit with offerings, which are sometimes recorded in the form of a list. When the time comes, the promise must be kept, under the threat of sanctions, which vary in severity according to the power of the spirit (ranging from illness to death). Communication between the spirits of the land and humans is established either through a medium possessed by a spirit which speaks through his mouth, or through dreams in which the *neak ta* usually sets out specific needs or desires. These are much the same as those of the living: drink, cigarettes, food, perfume....

Some mass graves, whether sites of massacres or simply wells into which corpses were thrown – including, it should be noted, corpses of Khmer Rouge cadres killed in purges – are thought by villagers to possess some of the same characteristics as the places where the tutelary spirits reside. For instance, a young teacher who took me to see a former killing field pointed out that some huge termite hills had grown up there. Now, termite hills are a symbol of the 'earth growing' and often indicate the presence of a chthonian spirit.[30] An even clearer example of this parallel between *neak ta* and the anonymous dead of the genocide was provided by a nearby site where an old well had been used as a mass grave in 1979.[31] Two women who lived nearby dreamed of this grave. The first, younger woman had a dream in which she saw a man dressed in black, most likely a Pol Potist,[32] who expressed his annoyance at the fact that, when she had come to pick fruits the day before, her foot had slipped on the edge of the well, causing a stone to fall in. The following day she atoned for the offence she had caused with an offering of incense, and was never subsequently troubled. The other woman dreamed of a winning lottery number, which she claimed had been revealed by one of the dead from this mass grave. She expressed her gratitude by building a small altar typical of the little dwellings of the *neak ta*, which are miniature versions of human houses.

However, alongside these sites considered as 'active', and which the villagers have integrated within their everyday existence, there are, it is important to note, other places which, although explicitly devoted to commemoration, are not assigned the same value by those living near them. One such is a memorial on the site of a former detention centre in the Samrong Knong monastery, not far from the town of Battambang; it was erected by Cambodians who fled as refugees to the United States and France.[33] This cement-built memorial contains dozens of skeletons, visible through windows, and has bas-relief sculptures showing the torture inflicted upon prisoners. A small pot of incense, clearly placed there some time ago, shows that people do not regularly leave offerings at this site. And according to those living nearby, this place is not 'active': no dreams, no nocturnal lights to speak of, no termite mounds, no illnesses after visiting the site or such like have been reported. Placed on a concrete plinth, the bones in this memorial are not mixed with the earth, and are not at one with it. Furthermore, the dead are not completely anonymous, as French and American Cambodians have recognized members of their families among them. These bodies are not 'earth-bodies', and thus do not fit into the system of interpretation based on Khmer religious beliefs.

Lastly, it is important to point out that these dreams establishing a link between the living and the 'earth-dead' of certain mass graves left by the Khmer Rouges occurred more than ten years after the toppling of the Democratic Kampuchea regime. Indeed, in one case the woman in question had no actual personal experience of this period, as she was born in the 1980s. This form of communication, occurring within a framework structured by Khmer religious beliefs, makes it possible for subsequent generations of the living to engage in a somewhat 'on–off' relationship with these 'earth-dead', according to the memory-centred needs of survivors. Furthermore, these 'earth-dead' may express different 'points of view' over time.

Notes

1 S. Breton (ed.), *Qu'est-ce qu'un corps?* (Paris: Musée du Quai Branly-Flammarion, 2004).
2 Khmers make up around 90 per cent of the population of Cambodia, referred to as a whole as Cambodians. The 'Khmer Rouges' were communist Khmers, nicknamed thus by Sihanouk in the 1950s.
3 R. Hertz, 'Contribution à une étude sur la représentation collective de la mort (1907)', in *Sociologie religieuse et folklore* (Paris: Presses Universitaires de France, 1970 – original edition 1928), pp. 14–80.
4 Democratic Kampuchea was the official name of the Khmer Rouge regime.
5 D. Fassin, *When Bodies Remember: Experience and Politics of AIDS in South Africa* (Berkeley: University of California Press, 2007 – original French edition 2006).
6 Not its real name.
7 The term 'spirit' is placed in inverted commas because it does not quite render the exact status of these beings.
8 The area between the forested plateau of the Cardamoms and Lake Tonle Sap.
9 My research was carried out in the former Khmer Rouge districts (*dambon*) numbers 2 and 7.
10 D. P. Chandler, *The Tragedy of Cambodian History: Politics, War, and Revolution Since 1945* (New Haven: Yale University Press, 1991), pp. 269–70.

11 There is an ongoing debate between Ben Kiernan and Steven Heder over the function of these Khmer scarves: the former sees the distribution of these identifying scarves as the first phase of a plan of extermination; the latter argues that, on the contrary, the extermination was not planned, even if the end result was the same, given that the Pol Pot regime 'inspired by a modernizing ideology with genocidal potentialities, realizes those potentialities through a set of genocidal practices'. I refer to this difference of opinion because it is representative of the debates surrounding the nature of the Khmer Rouge regime, debates which have only increased in intensity with the creation in 2007 of the Extraordinary Chambers in the Courts of Cambodia, in which various former leading figures from Democratic Kampuchea are standing trial. See B. Kiernan, *The Pol Pot Regime: Race, Power, and Genocide in Cambodia Under the Khmer Rouge, 1975–1979* (New Haven: Yale University Press, 1996); S. Heder, 'Racism, Marxism, labelling and genocide in Ben Kiernan's *The Pol Pot Regime*', *South East Asia Research*, 5:2 (1997), pp. 101–53.
12 I have examined this question in greater detail in A. Y. Guillou, 'Traces of destruction and thread of continuity in post-genocide Cambodia', in V. Das & C. Han (eds), *An Anthropology of Living and Dying in the Contemporary World* (Berkeley: California University Press, forthcoming).
13 R. Rechtman, 'L'empreinte des morts: remarques sur l'intentionnalité génocidaire', in S. Phay-Vakalis (ed.), *Cambodge, l'atelier de la mémoire* (Paris: Université Paris 8/Phnom Penh, Sonleuk Tmey-Centre Bophana, 2010), pp. 133–7.
14 The social groups holding differing perspectives on the genocide and how to deal with it are, respectively, Cambodia's ruling party, the Cambodian diaspora, the Khmer Rouge tribunal, Buddhist religious institutions, Cambodian villagers and the minority Cham Muslim population (who hold Cambodian nationality), who are today increasingly active.
15 In September 1981, the Khmer Rouges, the Son Sannists (non-communist nationalists) and the Sihanoukists created a coalition opposed to the pro-Vietnamese government in Phnom Penh. This coalition was given diplomatic recognition by western countries and the United Nations until the peace accords signed between the four Cambodian factions in 1991.
16 On these memorials and museums, see R. Hughes, *Fielding Genocide: Post-1979 Cambodia and the Geopolitics of Memory*, PhD thesis, University of Melbourne (2006); and J.-L. Margolin, 'L'Histoire brouillée: musées et mémoriaux du génocide cambodgien', *Gradhiva, Musée du Quai Branly*, 5 (2007), pp. 85–95.
17 Information provided by a villager from Bakan district who had taken part in the preparation of these bones in Phnom Penh.
18 Hughes, *Fielding Genocide*.
19 A. Y. Guillou, 'An alternative memory of the Khmer Rouge genocide: the dead of the mass graves and the land guardian spirits (*neak ta*)', *South East Asia Research*, 20:2 (2012), pp. 193–212.

20 I am grateful to Fabienne Luco, who made me aware of this point.
21 In Khmer thought, among the elements of which the human body is composed (water, wind, air, fire, earth), earth (*dey*) is associated with corpses. It is the last element that remains following death.
22 For example, the ceremonies for placing ritual markers in Buddhist monasteries (*banchoh seima*) are a rich source of ethnographic material regarding the element 'earth'.
23 I was nonetheless forced to carry out this sort of interview in some circumstances. I was, for example, more or less 'summoned' by a woman from Kompong Tralach who insisted on describing in detail what she had suffered under the Khmer Rouge regime, including the loss of her children, who one by one died of starvation. It was important for her to see her terrible, and utterly typical, account being written down in my notebook.
24 Psychiatrists working with Cambodian patients have also come up against the limitations of the individual interview. See G. Welsh, 'La tour de Babel: émergence d'une approche psychanalytique de groupe avec des réfugiés', *Revue Française de Psychanalyse*, 75:4 (2011), pp. 1139–50.
25 A. Y. Guillou, 'The living archeology of a painful heritage: the first and second life of the Khmer Rouge mass graves', in M. S. Falser & M. Juneja (eds), *'Archaeologizing' Heritage? Transcultural Entanglements Between Local Social Practices and Global Virtual Realities* (Heidelberg: Springer, 2013), pp. 259–69. The 'treasures' include Angkorean and post-Angkorean statues that pepper Cambodia's soil, Buddhist icons such as those found by Lady Penh in the foundation myth of the capital, Phnom Penh, the precious pottery buried in certain locations which, according to legend, reveals itself to human eyes in order that it might be 'borrowed'.
26 This expression has been identified by Fabienne Luco in his ongoing doctoral thesis in anthropology.
27 This old woman may have been a former Khmer Rouge low-rank cadre herself. I have not yet been able to verify this, however, because she lives in a different village from the one where I stay and where everybody knows each other.
28 C. Ang, *Les Êtres surnaturels dans la religion populaire khmère* (Paris: Cedoreck, 1986).
29 C. Ang, 'Le sol et l'ancêtre. L'amorphe et l'anthropomorphe', *Journal Asiatique*, 1:1 (1995), pp. 213–38, at p. 222.
30 This should be seen in parallel with the remarks made above regarding the dead making the earth 'grow'.
31 Guillou, 'An alternative memory'.
32 Khmer Rouge fighters and cadres wore black.
33 I am grateful to Sina Emde and Ute Luig of the Freie Universität, Berlin, for drawing my attention to this memorial.

Bibliography

Ang, C., *Les Êtres surnaturels dans la religion populaire khmère* (Paris: Cedoreck, 1986)

Ang, C., 'Le sol et l'ancêtre. L'amorphe et l'anthropomorphe', *Journal Asiatique*, 1:1 (1995), pp. 213–38

Breton, S. (ed.), *Qu'est-ce qu'un corps?* (Paris: Musée du Quai Branly-Flammarion, 2004)

Chandler, D. P., *The Tragedy of Cambodian History: Politics, War, and Revolution Since 1945* (New Haven: Yale University Press, 1991)

Fassin, D., *When Bodies Remember: Experience and Politics of AIDS in South Africa* (Berkeley: University of California Press, 2007 – original French edition 2006)

Guillou, A. Y., 'An alternative memory of the Khmer Rouge genocide: the dead of the mass graves and the land guardian spirits *(neak ta)*', *South East Asia Research*, 20:2 (2012), pp. 193–212

Guillou, A. Y, 'The living archeology of a painful heritage: the first and second life of the Khmer Rouge mass graves', in M. S. Falser & M. Juneja (eds), *'Archaeologizing' Heritage? Transcultural Entanglements Between Local Social Practices and Global Virtual Realities* (Heidelberg: Springer, 2013), pp. 259–69

Guillou, A. Y., 'Traces of destruction and thread of continuity in post-genocide Cambodia', in V. Das & C. Han (eds), *An Anthropology of Living and Dying in the Contemporary World* (Berkeley: California University Press, forthcoming)

Heder, S., 'Racism, Marxism, labelling and genocide in Ben Kiernan's *The Pol Pot Regime*', *South East Asia Research*, 5:2 (1997), pp. 101–53

Hertz, R., 'Contribution à une étude sur la représentation collective de la mort (1907)', in *Sociologie religieuse et folklore* (Paris: Presses Universitaires de France, 1970 – original edition 1928), pp. 14–80

Hughes, R., *Fielding Genocide: Post-1979 Cambodia and the Geopolitics of Memory*, PhD thesis, University of Melbourne (2006)

Kiernan, B., *The Pol Pot Regime: Race, Power, and Genocide in Cambodia Under the Khmer Rouge, 1975–1979* (New Haven: Yale University Press, 1996)

Margolin, J.-L., 'L'Histoire brouillée: musées et mémoriaux du génocide cambodgien', *Gradhiva, Musée du Quai Branly*, 5 (2007), pp. 85–95

Rechtman, R., 'L'empreinte des morts: remarques sur l'intentionnalité génocidaire', in S. Phay-Vakalis (ed.), *Cambodge, l'atelier de la mémoire* (Paris: Université Paris 8/Phnom Penh, Sonleuk Tmey-Centre Bophana, 2010), pp. 133–7

Welsh, G., 'La tour de Babel: émergence d'une approche psychanalytique de groupe avec des réfugiés', *Revue Française de Psychanalyse*, 75:4 (2011), pp. 1139–50

8
Display, concealment and 'culture': the disposal of bodies in the 1994 Rwandan genocide

Nigel Eltringham

Introduction

In their ethnography of violent conflict, 'cultures of terror'[1] and genocide, anthropologists have recognized that violence is discursive. The victim's body is a key vehicle of that discourse. In contexts of inter-ethnic violence, for example, ante-mortem degradation and/or post-mortem mutilation are employed to transform the victim's body into a representative example of the ethnic category, the manipulation of the body enabling the victimizer to materially actualize an otherwise abstract fantasy of alterity. Where research has focused on ultimate disposal, it has been in 'cultures of terror' where bodies are displayed and serve an instrumental and didactic role. While research has revealed commonalities in the discursive use of the body in such contexts, there has been less attention paid to contexts of *extermination*, where bodies are not called upon to play instrumental, didactic roles, but are concealed through burial (Srebrenica) or cremation (Auschwitz-Birkenau). If ante-mortem degradation and post-mortem mutilation in such contexts are to be understood as discursive practices drawing on cultural repertoires, is the manner in which the body is disposed of part of a continuum, or does it mark a disjuncture because the discursive potential of the body has been exhausted? Is the part the corpse plays in 'cultures of terror' absent from contexts of genocide because perpetrators *conceal* their intentions (from their victims and others) rather than communicate them through corpses?

In the case of the Rwandan genocide, the binary of concealment/ didactic display is insufficient, given that bodies were concealed (collected and buried); dumped in rivers; and left exposed where they were killed. Using Rwanda as a case study, this chapter proposes an agenda for ethnographic research to explore the relationship between concealment and display in contexts of genocide, with attention to the discursive quality of the disposal of bodies. This relationship is explored in detail after a discussion of the historical background to the 1994 genocide.

Context: the Rwandan genocide

While for the period prior to 1860, historians know virtually nothing about how the terms 'Hutu', 'Tutsi' and 'Twa' were used in social discourse,[2] we do know that the formation of pre-colonial Rwanda was driven by the expansion of a core central kingdom ruled by a *mwami* ('king') drawn from the *Bahindiro* Tutsi lineage of the *Nyiginya* clan.[3] 'Tutsi' originally referred to this elite of cattle herders: the *mwami* and his court. Around 1890, chiefs introduced a form of unpaid labour (*uburetwa*) requiring tenant farmers to work for the chief. This was required only of farmers, who, in response to a gradual extension of the term 'Tutsi' to all herders, became known as 'Hutu' (a term previously used to indicate non-elite farmers or cattle herders).[4] As a consequence, the paramount meaning of 'Tutsi' denoted proximity to the central court and 'proximity to power',[5] while 'Hutu', which had initially indicated 'social son, client, or someone who does not possess cattle',[6] 'came to be associated with and eventually defined by inferior status'.[7]

It was to the apex of this system, the court of the central kingdom, that colonial authorities came (German 1897–1916, Belgian 1916 onwards) and erroneously took the 'aristocrats of the Rwandan court to be the models of the "Tutsi" in general',[8] even though of 50,000 Tutsi men in Rwanda in 1900, only 2,500 (5 per cent) held any political authority, the rest being *'petits'* or *'non-élite* Tutsi'.[9]

The Belgian authorities (with a significant input from Roman Catholic missionaries) intensified the existing *process* of hierarchialization with a form of indirect rule that devolved new forms of power and wealth accumulation to the chiefs, accelerating the crystallization of social distinction begun at the end of the nineteenth century.[10] All of these *practical* changes were underpinned by a racial, social evolutionary ideology: the 'Hamitic hypothesis', which asserted that African 'civilization' was due to racially distinct 'Caucasoid' invaders from the north/north-east of Africa.[11]

The culmination of this process of *racialization* was the census of 1933–34, in which every Rwandan was assigned an 'ethno-racial' label (15 per cent Tutsi, 84 per cent Hutu, 1 per cent Twa) and issued with an ID card upon which the label was inscribed. Following patrilineal custom, children would inherit the identity inscribed on their father's ID card.[12] Until 1997, the French term *ethnie* and the Kinyarwanda term *ubwoko* appeared on the ID card. For the colonial authorities, both terms were 'synonyms for race in the biologically determinist sense'.[13]

As possible independence drew near, both a newly emergent Hutu elite (trained by the Roman Catholic Church) and the Tutsi court deployed the Hamitic hypothesis to argue, respectively, that the end of Belgian rule must also be the end of Tutsi rule, or that the Tutsi monarchy should remain in place.[14] And yet, at the end of the 1950s, the average family income of Hutu and *petits* Tutsi (90–97 per cent of those designated Tutsi) was virtually the same,[15] with only 10,000 élite Tutsi (out of 300,000 of those designated Tutsi) being associated with the political class[16] – a 'minority among their own people'.[17]

Two political parties were formed in 1959, the elite-Tutsi Union Nationale Rwandaise (UNAR) and the Parti du Mouvement de l'Emancipation Hutu (Parmehutu), the latter founded by Grégoire Kayibanda. In November 1959 violence sparked by the assault of a Parmehutu leader by UNAR activists led to further violence;[18] around 1,000 Tutsi were killed and around 10,000 Tutsi fled Rwanda.[19] By 14 November, Belgian authorities had restored order in favour of Parmehutu (known as the 'Social Revolution').[20] In July 1960, the renamed Mouvement Démocratique Républicain-Parmehutu (MDR-Parmehutu) won two-thirds of the vote in communal elections and, in January 1961, seized power (with the help of the Belgians), Kayibanda becoming Prime Minister. MDR-Parmehutu won a majority in parliamentary elections in September 1961, Kayibanda became President in October, and a referendum abolished the monarchy. Rwanda gained independence on 1 July 1962.

In 1960, Tutsi exiles, calling themselves *ingenzi* ('brave'), but called *inyenzi* ('cockroach') by opponents, began to launch raids. Following a raid in December 1963, Tutsi politicians were executed and 14,000 Tutsi massacred. By January 1964, some 336,000 Tutsi had taken refuge outside of Rwanda.[21]

By 1970, the government was dominated by people from Kayibanda's home area in central Rwanda. To deflect regional resentment, Kayibanda used the killing of 150,000 Hutu in Burundi in April 1972 by the Tutsi-dominated army to 'check' whether the 9 per cent quota for Tutsi was being 'respected' in the civil service and schools.[22] Unrest followed and Major-General Juvénal Habyarimana (from the north-west) seized power on 5 July 1973; declared himself President; created a new party in 1975, the Mouvement Révolutionnaire National pour le Développement (MRND);[23] and excluded Tutsi from public life. In 1987, Tutsi refugees formed the Rwandan Patriotic Front (RPF) with an armed wing, the Rwandan Patriotic Army (RPA).[24]

In a context of economic crisis, and after French President François Mitterand in June 1990 made development aid conditional on democratization, Habyarimana created a commission to investigate 'democratization'.[25] On 1 October, the RPA attacked from Uganda, but were repelled by the Rwandan army, the Forces Armées Rwandaises (FAR), who then proceeded to kill 1,500 Tutsi civilians.[26] A cease-fire was agreed in November.

In early 1991, the FAR murdered 1,000 Tutsi.[27] Following a new constitution (June 1991) opposition parties (demanding negotiations with the RPF) emerged, including the Mouvement Démocratique Républicain (MDR) and the multi-ethnic Parti Liberal (PL).[28] In March 1993, 300 Tutsi were killed by the Presidential Guard and *interahamwe* militia (see below) after the state radio (Radio Rwanda) claimed that the PL and RPF planned to assassinate opposition leaders.[29] The opposition parties, however, remained united and forced Habyarimana to form a coalition cabinet with opposition party members.[30] On 1 April 1992, the racist and exclusively Hutu Coalition pour la Défense de la République (CDR) was formed.

On 2 April 1992, Dismas Nsengiyaremye (of the MDR) became Prime Minister and began negotiations with the RPF at Arusha, Tanzania, leading to the 'Arusha Accords' (see below), key features of which were: the right of Tutsi refugees to return to Rwanda; the integration of the FAR and RPA; and a multi-party 'Broad-Based Transitional Government' (BBTG) which would incorporate the RPF.[31] Those in the MDR who had supported the negotiations with the RPF were denounced as traitors by anti-RPF elements of their own party who declared themselves 'MDR-Power'.[32]

On 8 July 1993, the extremist Radio Télévision Libre des Mille Collines (RTLM) began broadcasting. Propaganda maintained that the 'gains' of the 1959 'Social Revolution' (a state controlled by 'the Hutu') had to be protected from 'Tutsi feudalists' (RPF) who planned to exterminate Hutu assisted by Tutsi 'accomplices' (*ibyitso*).[33]

In August 1993 Habyarimana signed the Arusha Accords and in October the United Nations Security Council authorized 2,500 peacekeepers (the United Nations Assistance Mission for Rwanda, UNAMIR) to oversee the installation of the new multi-party government.[34] On 21 October, the recently elected President of Burundi, Melchior Ndadaye (a Hutu), was assassinated by Tutsi army officers.[35] Two days later, at an MDR-Power rally, Frodauld Karamira (second Vice-President of the MDR) rejected the Arusha Accords and declared that 'we have plans "to work"' (kill Tutsi).[36] In 1992 the Mouvement Républicain National pour la Démocratie et le Développement (MRND(D)) had formed the *Interahmwe* ('those who fight together') militia and in 1993 the CDR formed the *Impuzamugambi* militia ('those who have the same goal').[37] Both were given military training and arms by the Presidential Guard.

Returning to Kigali on 6 April 1994 from a conference in Dar-es-Salaam, Habyarimana's aircraft (also carrying President Ntaryamira of Burundi) was shot down by surface-to-air missiles, killing all on board. Although both Hutu extremists and the RPA have been accused of the attack,[38] a report by experts commissioned by a French judge concluded in 2012 that the missile was fired from a position held by the Presidential Guard.[39]

On 7 April 1994, three Hutu opposition party ministers, the Hutu Prime Minister and ten Belgian UN peacekeepers were murdered by the Presidential Guard (Belgium withdrew its UN troops on 13 April). As coordinated massacres of Tutsi spread, and the RPF launched a new offensive, an 'interim government' was created at meetings on 8 April (chaired by Colonel Théoneste Bagosora) and Jean Kambanda became Prime Minister.

Soldiers and police distributed arms and coordinated killing by militia and civilians. Mayors coordinated house-to-house searches and roadblocks. RTLM incited killing and revealed where Tutsi were hiding. Members of the interim government continually made broadcasts, calling for '*inyenzi*' and '*ibyitso*' to be killed. Tutsi (men, women and children) were killed with machetes, hoes, spears, hammers and nailed clubs, despite having sought safety at church and hospital complexes; because they appeared on a pre-written list; were personally known to their attackers; or because of ID cards.[40] Many Hutu refused to participate and/or hid Tutsi.[41] The 2001 census estimated 937,000 Rwandans were killed between April and July 1994, the vast majority Tutsi.⁴² In late 1994, a UN official alleged that the RPA alone had killed 25,000–45,000 Hutu in April–September that year.⁴³

The body as discursive vehicle

Anthropologists have argued that violence should be analysed as a 'discursive practice – whose symbols and rituals are as relevant to its enactment as its instrumental aspects'.⁴⁴ In other words, violence is a 'meaningful cultural expression' rather than 'the absence of and destruction of all cultural and social order'.⁴⁵ Mass violence, therefore, displays 'macabre forms of cultural design and violent predictability'.⁴⁶ This suggests that, in approaching episodes of genocide or mass violence, we must attend to the '"poetics" of violent practice', those context-specific dimensions of violence that are 'used discursively to amplify the cultural force of violent acts'.⁴⁷

The key vehicle for the articulation of this discourse is the body. Difference is manufactured, actualized and amplified by manipulating the body.⁴⁸ Discussing the Rwandan genocide, Christopher Taylor states that 'it is the human body that serves as the ultimate tablet upon which the dictates of the state are inscribed'.⁴⁹ Citing Kafka's *In the Penal Colony* (1919), Taylor suggests 'that societies "write" their signatures onto the bodies of their sacrificial victims'. As in Kafka's story of a machine that writes with needles on the condemned, so the *direct* inscription of the tattoo received by Primo Levi at Monowitz (a satellite camp of Auschwitz-Birkenau) is part of a wider process where difference is inscribed on a body, from the shaving of the head, to emaciation, to the 'unnatural hard gait' caused by 'repellent wooden shoes'.⁵⁰ Given that the perpetrator's fantasies do not correspond with members of the target group ordinarily encountered (see Zygment Bauman's distinction between the 'real' and 'conceptual' Jew⁵¹) particular forms of ante-mortem degradation, killing and/or post-mortem mutilation are required to 'stabilise the body of the ethnic other', to make tangible and concrete what is otherwise 'unstable and deceptive'.⁵² It is in this sense that the target is 'elusive' because 'the people one kills are never those one actually sees but merely what they represent, that is, what is hidden under their mask of innocence and normality'.⁵³ Corporal manipulation, therefore, 'removes' the mask, thereby producing 'abstract tokens' of a targeted group 'out of the bodies of real persons'.⁵⁴ As Lisa Malkki observes in the context of the 1972 genocide of Hutu in Burundi, it is 'through violence that bodies of individual persons become metamorphosed into specimens of the [category] for which they are supposed to stand'.[55] In other words, it is through ante-mortem degradation, particular forms of killing and/or post-mortem mutilation that 'categorical certainty' is achieved.[56] Genocidal violence is, therefore, not simply a matter of eliminating the ethnic other; rather, it 'involves the use of the body to establish the parameters of this otherness, taking the body apart to divine the enemy within'.[57] In the case of Auschwitz, for example, there had to be a 'demolition of a man' in order that the 'true' *Untermensch* (sub-human) could be 'unmasked'.[58] As Michael Taussig suggests, 'the victimizer needs the victim for the purpose of making truth, objectifying the victimizer's fantasies in the discourse of the other', where the key vehicle for the articulation of this discourse is the body of the other.[59]

This review of anthropological commentary suggests a consensus regarding the role of a victim's body ante-mortem in contexts of violent conflict, 'cultures of terror' and genocide. When the post-mortem disposal of bodies and their discursive role are considered, however, we encounter diversity. While genocide involves concealment of the dead (discursive/didactic potential is exhausted), violent conflict and 'cultures of terror' often involve display of the dead (discursive/didactic potential continues). The problem, though, is that not all contexts conform to this duality; not all cultures of terror involve display and not all genocides only involve concealment.

Regarding the didactic use of dead bodies in cultures of terror, María Victoria Uribe, writing on the context of *La Violencia* in Colombia in the 1950s (in which up to 300,000 people were killed), describes post-mortem 'semantic operations' which 'turned the victims into animals'.[60] As Uribe observes, '*La Violencia* wasn't simply about killing Others; their bodies had to be dismembered and transformed into something else'.[61] These post-mortem 'semantic procedures' (cuts made with a machete) had a particular cultural logic, relying on folk understandings of the analogy between animal and human physiology. Moreover, the terms used for these cuts were everyday terms used for butchering and the preparation of food, and drew on the way the peasants conceived of their own bodies.[62] These mutilated corpses were then used instrumentally, 'displayed in highly visible places' so that they became 'terrifying alterities, pedagogical and exemplifying texts that always achieved their objective' – to frighten inhabitants away.[63] Joost Fontein suggests that bodies used in this way possess a form of 'agency' in that they affect 'the living, provoking and structuring their responses' through what he terms their 'emotive materiality'.[64]

Deploying dead bodies as didactic objects is, of course, commonplace in 'cultures of terror'.[65] Regarding the comparative study of the disposal of bodies, this suggests a division between the instrumental, didactic display of bodies in 'cultures of terror', where the intention is to *discipline* a population, and, in contrast, the concealment of bodies in contexts of genocide, where the intention is to *exterminate* a population. And yet, this duality is insufficient. Not all 'cultures of terror' display dead bodies instrumentally.

Antonius Robben describes how during the 'Dirty War' in Argentina (1976–82) the military junta 'incinerated, dumped at sea or buried in mass graves' between 10,000 and 30,000 victims of the 'political left'.[66] As with the 'cultural logic' found in Uribe's Colombian example, so Robben suggests that the junta intentionally exploited a 'cultural complex' found in Argentina which requires 'general human care for the dead and the emotional need for mourning'. Although corpses were concealed, didactic terror was maintained, because disappearance struck at the 'very core of Argentine society', etching 'a silhouette in the homes of surviving family members'.[67] It was the absence, rather than the display, of the dead body that was instrumental.

While bodies can be displayed (Colombia) or concealed (Argentina), the case of political violence in Zimbabwe since 1999 demonstrates that both can be present. Joost Fontein notes that while some bodies of members of the opposition Movement for Democratic Change (MDC) were 'deliberately left in prominent places, along roads or pathways', other bodies were concealed in concrete-filled coffins thrown into dams and lakes.[68] Although Fontein implies that while the displayed bodies served the didactic role noted above,[69] the concealment of bodies and the disruption of MDC funerals were intentionally designed to disturb practices akin to the 'cultural complex' noted by Robben,[70] by preventing 'the material, social and symbolic processes and techniques through which things and substances become human remains, bodies become bones, and living people become safely dead'.[71] In the Zimbabwean context, both display *and* concealment served to transgress the normal processes of 'containment and transformation' of the dead.[72] Given that the examples of Argentina and Zimbabwe disrupt the supposed nexus of 'culture of terror'/display, does the case of Rwanda correspond to the supposed nexus of genocide/concealment?

Flows, concealment and exposure in the Rwandan genocide

Christopher Taylor[73] suggests, in the context of Rwanda, 'something political and historical happened in Rwanda in 1994, but something cultural happened as well.… Beneath the aspect of disorder there lay an eerie order to the violence.… Many of the actions followed a cultural patterning, a structured and structuring logic.'[74] In a sophisticated analysis drawing on his research into popular medicine in Rwanda and the cosmology of the pre-independence monarchy, Taylor[75] suggests that Rwandans[76] conceive of the body through a 'flow/blockage symbolism' (especially the orderly flow of fluids – milk, semen, blood) which 'mediates between physiological, sociological and cosmological levels of causality'.[77] Within this symbolism, 'unobstructed connection and unimpeded movement' are valued, but there is also an 'internal dialectic' that one cannot have 'flow' without 'blockage'.[78]

Taylor suggests that this 'flow/blockage' metaphor is apparent in the 1994 genocide,[79] that methods employed by the perpetrators 'betrayed a preoccupation with the movement of persons and substances and with the canals, arteries, and conduits along which persons and substances flow: rivers, roadways, pathways, and even the conduits of the human body such as the reproductive and digestive systems'.[80] In terms of the disposal of bodies, Taylor sees an expression of the flow metaphor in the dumping of bodies in the Nyabarongo and Akagera Rivers: 'Rwanda's rivers became part of the genocide by acting as the body politic's organs of elimination, in a sense "excreting" its hated internal other'.[81] At least 40,000 bodies were recovered from Lake Victoria, into which the Akagera River flows.[82] The dumping of bodies in these rivers has also been interpreted as an expression of the Hamitic hypothesis.[83] In a speech delivered on 22 November 1992, Léon Mugesera, Vice-President of the Gisenyi *préfecture* section of the ruling MRND(D), stated: 'Let me tell you that your home is Ethiopia and that we shall send you by the river Nyabarongo so that you'll get there quickly'.[84] We should note, however, that the propositions that the 'flow metaphor' and that the Hamitic hypothesis both influenced the disposal of bodies are speculative and neither has been substantiated with ethnographic research among perpetrators.

This way of disposal, with its (possible) discursive element(s), sits alongside a multiplicity of different ways in which dead bodies were treated during the 1994 genocide. Corpses were often left exposed where they were killed. When the journalist Fergal Keane arrived at Nyarubuye church (eighty-seven miles east of the capital, Kigali) the bodies remained where people had been killed three weeks earlier.[85] However, in the testimonies gathered by Omar McDoom[86] and Charles Mironko,[87] perpetrators indicate that victims were buried immediately. Then again, in the trial of Tharcisse Renzaho (*préfet* of Kigali-Ville during the genocide) at the International Criminal Tribunal for Rwanda (ICTR) eight witnesses (four prosecution and four defence) gave testimony that Renzaho had 'instructed truck and bulldozer drivers to dig holes and to collect bodies'.[88] According to one witness, 'Staff from the Red Cross, Ministry of Health, Ministry of Public Works and the prefecture's sanitation service participated in the clean-up operation'.[89] The Trial Chamber (the three judges) was indecisive regarding Renzaho's intention – public health or concealment:

> The Chamber observes that the removal of bodies from the streets of Kigali would certainly have the effect of improving the international community's impression of the situation. However, it would also have the effect of mitigating the public health risk. Therefore, concealment cannot be considered the only reasonable motive for the clean-up operation. The initiative and participation of the ICRC [International Committee of the Red Cross] in the task strengthen the notion that hygiene was a significant factor in the decision-making process.[90]

Ethnographic research may, of course, lead to different conclusions than that reached by the three judges, but this episode raises important questions. Was concealment the main reason for Renzaho's action, given that, where perpetrators were aware of the presence of UNAMIR soldiers, bodies were removed and burned?[91] Is the lack of concealment elsewhere (Nyarubuye for example) because these sites were distant from the capital and the international gaze, or is the lack of disposal in these sites simply due to a lack of authorities to implement such a policy and/or the absence of necessary equipment? Also, is 'public health', as the ICTR judgment implies, an 'acceptable' reason? Notions of disease, contamination, sanitizing and the need to protect 'public health' are prevalent euphemisms found in contexts of genocide.[92] To what extent is cleansing a town of the dead derivative from cleansing a town of the living?

These alternative interpretations revolve around the tension between intentional concealment versus 'public health'. However, studies of funeral rites in Rwanda and Rwandan attitudes to the dead raise even more complex possibilities. Claudine Vidal notes that it was only colonization and the introduction of Christianity to

Rwanda that introduced the practice of burial in cemeteries.[93] Prior to that, 'Rwandan culture ... was not interested in dead bodies'.[94] Rather, 'Immediately after death bodies, wrapped in a mat, were carried and abandoned in the forest, or buried near the house, and in the latter case, no sign marked the place of burial: neither grave nor ceremony'. Vidal[95] notes that the success of the Roman Catholic Church in Rwanda during Belgian colonization was more of a 'political than a religious victory'[96] and that 'a lot of "Christians", forced to display a façade of Christianity, clandestinely practised the religion of their ancestors'. According to Vidal, even those 'authentically Christianised' did not adopt western funereal practices wholeheartedly, and cemeteries were not considered special places.[97]

Additional detail provided by Gerard van't Spijker in his study of funeral rites in Rwanda suggests explanations for the diverse ways in which bodies were treated during the 1994 genocide.[98] Although van't Spijker indicates great diversity in the treatment of corpses in his study of funeral rites conducted in the 1980s, he describes a series of common post-mortem phases, one of which is *gushaka ishyamba*, the digging of the grave (commonly situated behind the deceased's house).[99] Vidal likewise states that 'the practice of burying the body in the family compound persists',[100] while other research reports that many genocide survivors favoured home burials and 'bemoaned the government's prohibition on private burials in the immediate vicinity of people's homes'.[101]

The significance of these insights for the treatment of bodies *during* the genocide is that the literal translation of *gushaka ishyamba* is 'look for a forest', which recalls the 'old custom of exposing the corpse in a non-cultivated place, forest or marsh'[102] or 'wild place'.[103] In pre-colonial Rwanda, the prevalence of burial or exposure was influenced by region and social status. Aléxis Kagame states that the Tutsi exposed their dead because they had a horror of decomposition and preferred to be 'eaten by hyenas' rather than worms, while in the north of the country, where the influence of the Tutsi central court was weaker, burial was more common.[104] Strangers who died in the north would, however, be thrown into the bush, a marsh, caves or even into holes.[105] If we compare these accounts with the disposal of bodies during the 1994 genocide, a series of questions present themselves, questions that can be answered only through ethnographic research. Were quick burials in compounds a form of concealment or a maintenance of funereal practice for those one had murdered? Were dead bodies left exposed simply because there was no need to conceal them, or was there some instrumental reference to *either* Tutsi as 'strangers' (the Hamitic hypothesis) or a mocking reference to pre-colonial/colonial practice in areas under the influence of the Tutsi central court? Rather than simply an indignity for the dead, were perpetrators re-enacting a symbolic 'ethnic' distinction from pre-independence Tutsi rule or an expression of Tutsi as 'Hamitic strangers'? Was exposure a symbolic reversal of the extremist media's description of Tutsi as 'hyenas who devour our children'?[106]

Conclusion

The suggestive questions posed in the last section are highly speculative and research may reveal that the disposal of bodies was more pragmatic, more a matter of the prosaic than the 'poetic'.[107] And yet, it remains the case that possible 'poetic', discursive elements of the disposal of bodies in contexts of genocide have been given insufficient attention. While this chapter has raised some tentative suggestions for research in the context of Rwanda, the discussion suggests that all contexts of genocide should be revisited and that the same attention should be paid to post-mortem disposal as has been given to ante-mortem degradation.

Notes

1 A 'culture of terror' is 'a relentless assault upon a civilian population in which menace, torture, forced labour and imprisonment become endemic forms of socio-political control'. J. A. Margold, 'From cultures of fear and terror to the normalisation of violence: an ethnographic case', *Critique of Anthropology*, 19:1 (1999), pp. 63–88, at p. 64. See also M. Taussig, 'Culture of terror – space of death: Roger Casement's Putumayo report and the explanation of torture', *Comparative Studies in Society and History*, 26:3 (1984), pp. 467–97.
2 J. Pottier, *Re-imagining Rwanda: Conflict, Survival and Disinformation in the Late Twentieth Century* (Cambridge: Cambridge University Press, 2002).
3 N. Eltringham, *Accounting for Horror: Post Genocide Debates in Rwanda* (London: Pluto Press, 2004), pp. 12–19; C. Newbury, 'Deux lignages au Kinyaga', *Cahiers d'Études Africaines*, 14:1 (1974), pp. 26–39; C. Newbury, 'Ethnicity in Rwanda: the case of Kinyaga', *Africa*, 48:1 (1978), pp. 17–29; C. Newbury, *The Cohesion of Oppression: Clientship and Ethnicity in Rwanda, 1860–1960* (New York: Colombia University Press, 1988), pp. 85ff.; D. Newbury, 'Understanding genocide', *African Studies Review*, 41:1 (1998), pp. 73–97.

4 J. Vansina, *Antecedents to Modern Rwanda: The Nyiginya Kingdom* (Oxford: James Currey, 2004), pp. 134–9.
5 Newbury, *The Cohesion of Oppression*, p. 51; J. Kagabo & V. Mudandagizi, 'Complainte des gens de l'argile', *Cahiers d'Études Africaines*, 14:53 (1974), pp. 75–87, at p. 76.
6 I. Jacob, *Dictionnaire Rwandais-Français: extrait du dictionnaire de l'Institut National de Recherche Scientifique* (Kigali: L'Imprimerie Scolaire, 1984), p. 590. Translations here and below from the French by the author.
7 Newbury, 'Ethnicity in Rwandaa', p. 21.
8 J.-P. Chrétien, 'Hutu et Tutsi au Rwanda et au Burundi', in J.-L. Amselle & E. M'Bokolo (eds), *Au coeur de l'ethnie: ethnies, tribalisme et état en Afrique* (Paris: Éditions la Découverte, 1985), p. 137.
9 I. Linden, *Church and Revolution in Rwanda* (Manchester: Manchester University Press, 1977), p. 18.
10 See Eltringham, *Accounting for Horror*, p. 15.
11 N. Eltringham, '"Invaders who have stolen the country": the Hamitic hypothesis, race and the Rwandan genocide', *Social Identities*, 12:4 (2006), pp. 425–46.
12 J.-P. Chrétien, J. F. Dupaquier, M. Kabanda & J. Ngarambe with Reporters Sans Frontiers (eds), *Rwanda: les médias du génocide* (Paris: Éditions Karthala, 1995), p. 161.
13 C. C. Taylor, *Sacrifice as Terror: The Rwandan Genocide of 1994* (Oxford: Berg, 1999), p. 62.
14 See Eltringham, 'Invaders who have stolen the country', pp. 433–5; F. Nkundabagenzi, *Rwanda Politique* (Brussels: Centre de Recherche de d'Information Socio-Politiques, 1961), pp. 22–8, 35–6.
15 Linden, *Church and Revolution*, p. 226.
16 J.-P. Harroy, *Rwanda: de la féodalité à la démocratie* (Souvenir d'un compagnon de la marche du Rwanda vers la démocratie et l'independance) (Brussels: Hayez, 1984), p. 234; H. Codere, *The Biography of an African Society: Rwanda 1900–1960: Based on Forty-Eight Rwandan Biographies* (Tervuren: Musée Royal de l'Afrique Central, 1973); A. Appadurai, 'Dead certainty: ethnic violence in the era of globalization', *Development and Change*, 29:4 (1998), pp. 905–25, at p. 20.
17 G. Prunier, *The Rwanda Crisis: History of a Genocide* (New York: Columbia University Press, 1995), n. 72.
18 Linden, *Church and Revolution*, p. 271.
19 F. Reyntjens, *L'Afrique des Grands Lacs en crise Rwanda–Burundi 1988–1994* (Paris: Karthala, 1994), p. 27.
20 See Eltringham, *Accounting for Horror*, p. 40.
21 Ibid., pp. 42–4.
22 F. Reyntjens, *Pouvoir et droit au Rwanda droit public et évolution politique 1916–1973* (Brussels: Musée Royal de l'Afrique Centrale, 1985), pp. 502–3.
23 Renamed Mouvement Républicain National pour la Démocratie et le Développement, MRND(D) in April 1991; see Eltringham, *Accounting for Horror*.

24 W. Cyrus-Reed, 'Exile, reform, and the rise of the Rwandan Patriotic Front', *Journal of Modern African Studies*, 34:3 (1996), pp. 479–501; M. Dorsey, 'Violence and power-building in post genocide Rwanda', in R. Doom & J. Gorus (eds), *Politics of Identity and Economics of Conflict in the Great Lakes Region* (Brussels: VUB University Press, 2000), pp. 311–48; G. Prunier, 'Eléments pour une histoire du Front patriote Rwandais', *Politique Africaine*, 51 (1993), pp. 121–38.
25 Chrétien *et al.*, *Rwanda*, p. 28.
26 Reyntjens, *L'Afrique des Grands Lacs*, pp. 94–6.
27 See Chrétien *et al.*, *Rwanda*, pp. 175–9.
28 See Eltringham, *Accounting for Horror*, pp. 78–9.
29 A. Guichaoua (ed.), *Les Crises politiques au Burindi et au Rwanda (1993–1994): analyses, faits, et documents* (Paris: Éditions Karthala, 1995), pp. 611–14.
30 J. Bertrand, *Le Rwanda, le piège de l'histoire: l'échec de l'opposition démocratique (1990–1994)* (Paris: Karthala, 2000).
31 See Eltringham, *Accounting for Horror*, pp. 84–5.
32 Ibid., pp. 88–9.
33 A. Des Forges, *'Leave None to Tell the Story': Genocide in Rwanda* (New York: Human Rights Watch, 1999), p. 78; Chrétien *et al.*, *Rwanda*.
34 M. Barnett, *Eyewitness to a Genocide: The United Nations and Rwanda* (Ithaca: Cornell University Press, 2002); R. A. Dallaire & B. Beardsley, *Shake Hands with the Devil: The Failure of Humanity in Rwanda* (Toronto: Random House Canada, 2003).
35 See Prunier, *The Rwanda Crisis*, p. 199.
36 Bertrand, *Le Rwanda*, p. 247; see also Des Forges, *'Leave None to Tell the Story'*, p. 138.
37 Des Forges, *'Leave None to Tell the Story'*, pp. 106ff.
38 See Eltringham, *Accounting for Horror*, pp. 111–18.
39 C. Oosterlinck, D. Van Schendel, J. Huon, J. Sompayrac & O. Chavanis, *Rapport d'expertise: destruction en vol du Falcon 50 Kigali (Rwanda)* (Paris: Cour d'appel de Paris Tribunal de Grande Instance de Paris, 2012).
40 See Des Forges *'Leave None to Tell the Story'*; L. A. Fujii, *Killing Neighbours: Webs of Violence in Rwanda* (Ithaca: Cornell University Press, 2009); J. Hatzfeld, *A Time for Machetes. The Rwandan Genocide: The Killers Speak* (London: Serpent's Tail, 2005); S. Straus, *The Order of Genocide: Race, Power, and War in Rwanda* (Ithaca: Cornell University Press, 2008).
41 African Rights, *Rwanda: Tribute to Courage* (London: African Rights, 2002).
42 IRIN (Integrated Regional Information Network for Central and Eastern Africa), 'Government puts genocide victims at 1.07 million', 19 December 2001, at www.irinnews.org/report/29236/rwanda-government-puts-genocide-victims-at-1-07-million (accessed 6 June 2014).
43 ICTR, Military I – Defence Exhibit DK112 – UN code cable, 'The "Gersoni" report Rwanda', admitted as evidence 16 November 2006,

para. 5. See also S. M. Khan, *The Shallow Graves of Rwanda* (London: I. B. Tauris, 2000), pp. 51–4.
44 N. L. Whitehead, 'Violence and the cultural order', *Daedalus*, 136:1 (2007), pp. 40–50, at pp. 40–4.
45 Ibid., p. 41.
46 Appadurai, 'Dead certainty', p. 909.
47 Whitehead, 'Violence and the cultural order', p. 45; Taussig, 'Culture of terror', p. 495.
48 A. L. Hinton, 'Why did the Nazis kill? Anthropology, genocide and the Goldhagen controversy', *Anthropology Today*, 14:5 (1998), pp. 9–15, at p. 14.
49 Taylor, *Sacrifice as Terror*, pp. 127–46.
50 P. Levi, *If This Is a Man; and, The Truce* (trans. S. J. Woolf) (London: Abacus, 2005 – original edition 1979), pp. 28–43.
51 Z. Bauman, *Modernity and the Holocaust* (Ithaca: Cornell University Press, 1991), pp. 38–9.
52 Appadurai, 'Dead certainty', p. 911.
53 O. Bartov, 'Defining enemies, making victims: Germans, Jews, and the Holocaust', *American Historical Review*, 103:3 (1998), pp. 771–816, at p. 785; see also Eltringham, *Accounting for Horror*, pp. 23–6; and 'Invaders who have stolen the country', p. 437.
54 Appadurai, 'Dead certainty', p. 920.
55 L. Malkki, *Purity and Exile: Violence, Memory and National Cosmology Among Hutu Refugees in Tanzania* (Chicago: University of Chicago Press, 1995), p. 910.
56 Appadurai, 'Dead certainty', p. 911.
57 Ibid., p. 913.
58 Levi, *If This Is a Man*, p. 28.
59 Taussig, 'Culture of terror', p. 469.
60 M. V. Uribe, 'Dismembering and expelling: semantics of political terror in Colombia', *Public Culture*, 16:1 (2004), pp. 79–95, at pp. 88–9.
61 Ibid., p. 88.
62 Ibid., p. 87.
63 Ibid., p. 89.
64 J. Fontein, 'Between tortured bodies and resurfacing bones: the politics of the dead in Zimbabwe', *Journal of Material Culture*, 15:4 (2010), pp. 423–48, at p. 432.
65 J. Zur, *Violent Memories: Mayan War Widows in Guatemala* (Boulder: Westview Press, 1998), p. 79.
66 A. C. G. M. Robben, 'State terror in the netherworld: disappearance and reburial in Argentina', in A. C. G. M. Robben (ed.), *Death, Mourning, and Burial: A Cross-Cultural Reader* (Oxford: Blackwell, 2004), p. 135.
67 Ibid., p. 137.
68 Fontein, 'Between tortured bodies', p. 434.
69 Ibid., p. 439.
70 Robben, 'State terror in the netherworld', p. 137.
71 Fontein, 'Between tortured bodies', p. 439.
72 Ibid., p. 437.

73 Taylor, *Sacrifice as Terror*, p. 101.
74 Ibid., pp. 102, 142-4. Taylor emphasizes, however, that the genocide was not 'caused' by Rwandan culture. On what Taylor understands 'culture' to mean, see ibid., pp. 99-102.
75 Ibid., pp. 110-26.
76 Ibid., pp. 112, 116; Taylor is cautious about claiming universal adherence or that the model is a 'fully conscious one'.
77 Ibid., pp. 111-12.
78 Ibid., pp. 125-6.
79 According to Taylor, ibid., p. 101, the Rwandan genocide 'in many respects was a massive ritual of purification, a ritual intended to purge the nation of "obstructing beings" as the threat of obstruction was imagined through a Rwandan ontology that situates the body politic in analogous relation to the individual human body'.
80 Ibid., p. 128.
81 Ibid., p. 130.
82 Dallaire & Beardsley, *Shake Hands with the Devil*, p. 336.
83 J. Meierhenrich, 'The transformation of lieux de mémoire: the Nyabarongo River in Rwanda, 1992-2009', *Anthropology Today*, 25:5 (2009), pp. 13-19.
84 Judgment in *The Canadian Minister of Citizenship and Immigration vs Léon Mugesera (and others)*, 8 September 2003. Author's translation from a French translation by Thomas Kamanzi.
85 F. Keane, *Season of Blood: A Rwandan Journey* (London: Viking, 1995), pp. 73-93.
86 O. McDoom, *Rwanda's Ordinary Killers: Interpreting Popular Participation in the Rwandan Genocide* (London: London School of Economics and Political Science, 2005), p. 5.
87 C. Mironko, 'Igitero: means and motive in the Rwandan genocide', *Journal of Genocide Research*, 6:1 (2004), pp. 47-60, at pp. 53-5.
88 ICTR, *The Prosecutor v. Tharcisse Renzaho*, Case no. ICTR-97-31-T, Judgment and sentence, 14 July 2009, para. 327.
89 Ibid., para. 328.
90 Ibid., para. 342.
91 Dallaire & Beardsley, *Shake Hands with the Devil*, p. 281.
92 B. Lang, *Act and Idea in the Nazi Genocide* (Chicago: University of Chicago Press, 1990), p. 16, n. 13.
93 C. Vidal, 'Le commémoration du génocide au Rwanda: violence symbolique, mémorisation forcée et histoire officielle', *Cahiers d'Études Africaines*, 44:3 (2004), pp. 575-92, at p. 578; see also M. d'Hertefelt, *Les Anciens royaumes de la zone interlacustre meridionale (Rwanda, Burundi, Buha* (London: International African Institute, 1962), p. 95.
94 Vidal, 'Le commémoration du génocide'.
95 Ibid., p. 579.
96 See T. Gatwa, *The Churches and Ethnic Ideology in the Rwandan Crises 1900-1994* (Regnum Studies in Mission) (Milton Keynes: Authentic Media, 2005); Linden, *Church and Revolution*; I. Linden, *Christianisme et pouvoirs au Rwanda, 1900-1990* (Paris: Karthala, 1999).

97 Vidal, 'Le commémoration du génocide', p. 579.
98 G. van't Spijker, *Les Usages funeraires et la mission de l'Eglise: une etude anthropologique et theologique des rites funeraires au Rwanda* (Kampen: Kok, 1990).
99 Ibid., p. 39.
100 Vidal, 'Le commémoration du génocide', p. 578.
101 J. Meierhenrich, 'Topographies of remembering and forgetting: the transformation of lieux de mémoire in Rwanda', in S. Straus & L. Waldorf (eds), *Remaking Rwanda: State Building and Human Rights After Mass Violence* (Madison: University of Wisconsin Press, 2011), pp. 283–96, p. 290; R. Ibreck, 'The politics of mourning: survivor contributions to memorials in post-genocide Rwanda', *Memory Studies*, 3:4 (2010), pp. 330–43, at p. 334.
102 van't Spijker, *Les Usages funeraires*, p. 61.
103 Vidal, 'Le commémoration du génocide', p. 578.
104 A. Kagame, *Les Organisations socio-familiales de l'Ancien Rwanda* (Brussels: Académie Royale des Sciences Coloniales, Classe des Sciences Morales et Politiques, 1954), p. 307.
105 van't Spijker, *Les Usages funeraires*, 93.
106 Chrétien *et al.*, *Rwanda*, p. 185.
107 Whitehead, 'Violence and the cultural order', p. 45.

Bibliography

African Rights, *Rwanda: Tribute to Courage* (London: African Rights, 2002)
Appadurai, A., 'Dead certainty: ethnic violence in the era of globalization', *Development and Change*, 29:4 (1998), pp. 905–25
Barnett, M., *Eyewitness to a Genocide: The United Nations and Rwanda* (Ithaca: Cornell University Press, 2002)
Bartov, O., 'Defining enemies, making victims: Germans, Jews, and the Holocaust', *American Historical Review*, 103:3 (1998), pp. 771–816
Bauman, Z., *Modernity and the Holocaust* (Ithaca: Cornell University Press, 1991)
Bertrand, J., *Le Rwanda, le piège de l'histoire: l'échec de l'opposition démocratique (1990-1994)* (Paris: Karthala, 2000)
Chrétien, J.-P., 'Hutu et Tutsi au Rwanda et au Burundi', in J.-L. Amselle & E. M'Bokolo (eds), *Au coeur de l'ethnie: ethnies, tribalisme et état en Afrique* (Paris: Éditions la Découverte, 1985), pp. 129–65
Chrétien, J.-P., J. F. Dupaquier, M. Kabanda & J. Ngarambe with Reporters Sans Frontiers (eds), *Rwanda: les médias du génocide* (Paris: Éditions Karthala, 1995)
Codere, H., *The Biography of an African Society: Rwanda 1900-1960: Based on Forty-Eight Rwandan Biographies* (Tervuren: Musée Royal de l'Afrique Central, 1973)
Cyrus-Reed, W., 'Exile, reform, and the rise of the Rwandan Patriotic Front', *Journal of Modern African Studies*, 34:3 (1996), pp. 479–501

Dallaire, R. A. & B. Beardsley, *Shake Hands with the Devil: The Failure of Humanity in Rwanda* (Toronto: Random House Canada, 2003)
Des Forges, A., *'Leave None to Tell the Story': Genocide in Rwanda* (New York: Human Rights Watch, 1999)
d'Hertefelt, M., *Les Anciens royaumes de la zone interlacustre méridionale (Rwanda, Burundi, Buha)* (London: International African Institute, 1962)
Dorsey, M., 'Violence and power-building in post genocide Rwanda', in R. Doom & J. Gorus (eds), *Politics of Identity and Economics of Conflict in the Great Lakes Region* (Brussels: VUB University Press, 2000), pp. 311–48
Eltringham, N., *Accounting for Horror: Post Genocide Debates in Rwanda* (London: Pluto Press, 2004)
Eltringham, N., '"Invaders who have stolen the country": the Hamitic hypothesis, race and the Rwandan genocide', *Social Identities*, 12:4 (2006), pp. 425–46
Fontein, J., 'Between tortured bodies and resurfacing bones: the politics of the dead in Zimbabwe', *Journal of Material Culture*, 15:4 (2010), pp. 423–48
Fujii, L. A., *Killing Neighbours: Webs of Violence in Rwanda* (Ithaca: Cornell University Press, 2009)
Gatwa, T., *The Churches and Ethnic Ideology in the Rwandan Crises 1900–1994* (Regnum Studies in Mission) (Milton Keynes: Authentic Media, 2005)
Guichaoua, A. (ed.), *Les Crises politiques au Burindi et au Rwanda (1993–1994): analyses, faits, et documents* (Paris: Éditions Karthala, 1995)
Harroy, J.-P., *Rwanda: de la féodalité à la démocratie* (Souvenir d'un compagnon de la marche du Rwanda vers la démocratie et l'independance) (Brussels: Hayez, 1984)
Hatzfeld, J., *A Time for Machetes. The Rwandan Genocide: The Killers Speak* (London: Serpent's Tail, 2005)
Hinton, A. L., 'Why did the Nazis kill? Anthropology, genocide and the Goldhagen controversy', *Anthropology Today*, 14:5 (1998), pp. 9–15
Ibreck, R., 'The politics of mourning: survivor contributions to memorials in post-genocide Rwanda', *Memory Studies*, 3:4 (2010), pp. 330–43
ICTR, Military I – Defence Exhibit DK112 – UN code cable, 'The "Gersoni" report Rwanda', admitted as evidence 16 November 2006
ICTR, *The Prosecutor v. Tharcisse Renzaho*, Case no. ICTR-97-31-T, Judgment and sentence, 14 July 2009
IRIN (Integrated Regional Information Network for Central and Eastern Africa), 'Government puts genocide victims at 1.07 million', 19 December 2001, at www.irinnews.org/report/29236/rwanda-government-puts-genocide-victims-at-1-07-million
Jacob, I., *Dictionnaire Rwandais-Français: extrait du dictionnaire de l'Institut National de Recherche Scientifique* (Kigali: L'Imprimerie Scolaire, 1984)
Kagabo, J. & V. Mudandagizi, 'Complainte des gens de l'argile', *Cahiers d'Études Africaines*, 14:53 (1974), pp. 75–87

Kagame, A., *Les Organisations socio-familiales de l'Ancien Rwanda* (Brussels: Académie Royale des Sciences Coloniales, Classe des Sciences Morales et Politiques, 1954)

Keane, F., *Season of Blood: A Rwandan Journey* (London: Viking, 1995)

Khan, S. M., *The Shallow Graves of Rwanda* (London: I. B. Tauris, 2000)

Lang, B., *Act and Idea in the Nazi Genocide* (Chicago: University of Chicago Press, 1990)

Levi, P., *If This Is a Man; and, The Truce* (trans. S. J. Woolf) (London: Abacus, 2005 – original edition 1979)

Linden, I., *Christianisme et pouvoirs au Rwanda, 1900–1990* (Paris: Karthala, 1999)

Linden, I., *Church and Revolution in Rwanda* (Manchester: Manchester University Press, 1977)

Malkki, L., *Purity and Exile: Violence, Memory and National Cosmology Among Hutu Refugees in Tanzania* (Chicago: University of Chicago Press, 1995)

Margold, J. A., 'From cultures of fear and terror to the normalisation of violence: an ethnographic case', *Critique of Anthropology*, 19:1 (1999), pp. 63–88

McDoom, O., *Rwanda's Ordinary Killers: Interpreting Popular Participation in the Rwandan Genocide* (London: London School of Economics and Political Science, 2005)

Meierhenrich, J., 'The transformation of lieux de mémoire: the Nyabarongo River in Rwanda, 1992–2009', *Anthropology Today*, 25:5 (2009), pp. 13–19

Meierhenrich, J., 'Topographies of remembering and forgetting: the transformation of lieux de mémoire in Rwanda', in S. Straus & L. Waldorf (eds), *Remaking Rwanda: State Building and Human Rights After Mass Violence* (Madison: University of Wisconsin Press, 2011), pp. 283–96

Mironko, C., '*Igitero*: means and motive in the Rwandan genocide', *Journal of Genocide Research*, 6:1 (2004), pp. 47–60

Newbury, C., 'Deux lignages au Kinyaga', *Cahiers d'Études Africaines*, 14:1 (1974), pp. 26–39

Newbury, C., 'Ethnicity in Rwanda: the case of Kinyaga', *Africa*, 48:1 (1978), pp. 17–29

Newbury, C., *The Cohesion of Oppression: Clientship and Ethnicity in Rwanda, 1860–1960* (New York: Colombia University Press, 1988)

Newbury, D., 'Understanding genocide', *African Studies Review*, 41:1 (1998), pp. 73–97

Nkundabagenzi, F., *Rwanda Politique* (Brussels: Centre de Recherche de d'Information Socio-Politiques, 1961)

Oosterlinck, C., D. Van Schendel, J. Huon, J. Sompayrac & O. Chavanis, *Rapport d'expertise: destruction en vol du Falcon 50 Kigali (Rwanda)* (Paris: Cour d'appel de Paris Tribunal de Grande Instance de Paris, 2012)

Pottier, J., *Re-imagining Rwanda: Conflict, Survival and Disinformation in the Late Twentieth Century* (Cambridge: Cambridge University Press, 2002)

Prunier, G., 'Eléments pour une histoire du Front patriote Rwandais', *Politique Africaine*, 51 (1993), pp. 121–38
Prunier, G., *The Rwanda Crisis: History of a Genocide* (New York: Columbia University Press, 1995)
Reyntjens, F., *L'Afrique des Grands Lacs en crise Rwanda–Burundi 1988–1994* (Paris: Karthala, 1994)
Reyntjens, F., *Pouvoir et droit au Rwanda: droit public et évolution politique 1916–1973* (Brussels: Musée Royal de l'Afrique Centrale, 1985)
Robben, A. C. G. M., 'State terror in the netherworld: disappearance and reburial in Argentina', in A. C. G. M. Robben (ed.), *Death, Mourning, and Burial: A Cross-Cultural Reader* (Oxford: Blackwell, 2004), pp. 134–48
Straus, S., *The Order of Genocide: Race, Power, and War in Rwanda* (Ithaca: Cornell University Press, 2008)
Taussig, M., 'Culture of terror – space of death: Roger Casement's Putumayo report and the explanation of torture', *Comparative Studies in Society and History*, 26:3 (1984), pp. 467–97
Taylor, C. C., *Sacrifice as Terror: The Rwandan Genocide of 1994* (Oxford: Berg, 1999)
Uribe, M. V., 'Dismembering and expelling: semantics of political terror in Colombia', *Public Culture*, 16:1 (2004), pp. 79–95
Vansina, J., *Antecedents to Modern Rwanda: The Nyiginya Kingdom* (Oxford: James Currey, 2004)
van't Spijker, *Les Usages funeraires et la mission de l'Eglise: une etude anthropologique et theologique des rites funeraires au Rwanda* (Kampen: Kok, 1990)
Vidal, C., 'Le commémoration du génocide au Rwanda: violence symbolique, mémorisation forcée et histoire officielle', *Cahiers d'Etudes Africaines*, 44:3 (2004), pp. 575–92
Whitehead, N. L., 'Violence and the cultural order', *Daedalus*, 136:1 (2007), pp. 40–50
Zur, J., *Violent Memories: Mayan War Widows in Guatemala* (Boulder: Westview Press, 1998)

9

An anthropological approach to human remains from the gulags

Élisabeth Anstett

We owe respect to the living
To the dead we owe only the truth.
(Voltaire)

Introduction

Archaeologists and anthropologists specializing in the field of funerary customs have long been used to considering the degree of social, religious and political investment placed in the dead body. Ever since the pioneering work of Robert Hertz, we have known that the social treatment of corpses is based on a series of rituals that bring into play the full range of collective representations relating to the perpetuation of the group.[1] These rituals frequently involve the use of temporary graves, as the final burial or cremation of the bodies is, in the societies studied by Hertz and in others, only the last stage of this process.

Few studies in this field, however, have dealt with collective burials. Anthropologists interested in the specific contexts of wars and epidemics[2] have developed the notion of 'catastrophe burial', which relates to the simultaneous mass burial of large numbers of corpses as a result of natural disasters, famine, disease or conflict.[3] Yet, up until very recently, the treatment of the bodies resulting from mass violence – or, for that matter, this extreme violence itself – has received little attention from anthropologists.[4]

However, a shift began with the large-scale exhumations undertaken in Bosnia and Spain, which shed new light on the fate of bodies in such situations and led anthropologists to consider the agendas underpinning a set of practices which, in a real sense, link the killers to their victims even after the death of the latter, and which are consequently all the more revealing of the processes governing the entry into – and exit from – violence. Studies such as those of Francisco Ferrandiz on Spain[5] and Elisabeth Claverie on Bosnia[6] have thus focused on the fate of the dead after their death, seeking to reveal by whom, how and exactly when the corpses were destroyed, buried, hidden or, on the contrary, displayed to the living/survivors. In so doing, these studies have revealed that the legal and symbolic status given to human remains in situations of mass violence can vary enormously, from that of material evidence to that of simple detritus. In this respect, the example of the violence perpetrated in the Soviet period is particularly revealing in a number of ways.

A long-lived and lethal institution

It is important to note from the outset that the deployment of violence through the gulag occurred on a historical, geographical and sociological scale that has rarely been equalled. The concentration camps which were first set up in the early months of the Bolshevik regime and subsequently spread across Russia and throughout the USSR would imprison, over the seventy years of their existence, around 15 million people. The precise nature of these camps, which were placed between 1930 and 1956 under the aegis of a dedicated central administration, the gulag,[7] varied greatly according to specific local situations and prevailing historical circumstances, as these factors largely dictated the living conditions (and therefore life expectancy) of detainees, depending on whether, for example, they were employed in the agricultural or industrial sectors, or in mining, or imprisoned during particularly harsh periods of famine or war.[8]

The stated aim of this dedicated central administration was to correct deviant minds through processes of deportation, incarceration and forced labour which made use of terror and extreme violence at every stage, with the objective, it must be emphasized, not of destroying the detainees, but rather of re-educating them.[9] For in the gulag, the physical and psychological enslavement of human beings was seen above all as a means of correction, albeit involving the death by exhaustion of the recalcitrant and the weak. In the camps, the wearing down of the body through work and hunger was the main tool[10] of 'correction' (*ispravlenie*), taken here to mean re-education. This said, the gulag was always a polymorphous and shifting institution whose boundaries were difficult to locate. It remains an object without any easily defined borders or contours.

An object with no clear beginning or end

Any attempt to locate the precise beginning and end of the gulag system thus faces considerable difficulties. Should 7 April 1930, the date of the decree by the Politburo setting up a central administration devoted to the running of the 're-education through labour' camps scheme, be taken as the date of the birth of the Soviet concentration camp system? Or should we consider that the latter began with the readiness, stated as early as January 1918, to use deportation, internment in concentration camps and forced labour as the principal means of dealing with political opposition?[11] What we can be sure of is that this rapidly established and long-lived coexistence of spaces of detention controlled by the state security organs alongside, and on the margins of, a prison system answering to the courts, constitutes the primary distinguishing feature of the gulag system.[12]

Similarly, should the end of the system be seen as occurring with the dismantling of the general administration of the camps at the end of 1956, or only with the large-scale release of dissidents by M. Gorbachev in 1986, which marked the end of this political instrumentalization of criminal justice and medicine? For a focus on the Stalinist period alone necessarily tends to neglect the question of the extraordinary longevity of the gulag system and, more generally, of the continuing practice, throughout the Soviet period, of sentencing individuals to deportation, internal exile and forced labour. The issue of the highly porous nature of the spaces of the gulags also needs to be addressed.

The stereotypical image of the camps as physically isolated and cut off from society[13] masks the true size of the net cast by these spaces, a net spread all the wider owing to the use of the gulags for large-scale civil engineering works from the 1920s onwards. This Soviet system can for this reason truly be said to cover the entirety of the territory of the former USSR.[14] The economic exploitation of the Soviet concentration camps thus helped to weave the gulags into the most ordinary spaces of everyday life: factories and hospitals, universities and residential buildings, roads and canals, mines, forests and farms.[15] Any part of the territory of the former USSR is liable to harbour traces of this aspect of the country's past. The high degree of communication between these places of detention and the rural and peri-urban locations of the industrial or agricultural installations to which detainees were led daily under escort was another enduring characteristic of the areas surrounding the camps, making an exhaustive cartography of the gulags virtually impossible.

The question of the social groups affected by the gulags is more complex still, given the successive generations of protagonists involved in a sprawling system which existed in a multitude of forms arguably from the beginning of the 1920s to the end of the 1980s. The estimated total number of people incarcerated therefore varies from around 10 to up to 20 million, according to the period under consideration, the particular courts and legislation involved, and the type of sentences in question.[16] However, after long years of controversy, and based on the most recent research, historians are now in general agreement that the gulag system caused the death of around 2 million people, a figure to which must be added the 800,000 murdered by the Soviet regime during the great purges.[17] Unlike the Nazi extermination camps, the history and sociology of which have been the subject of considerable amounts of research, a thorough sociological study of the gulag system has yet to be conducted. This is due in no small part to the difficulties involved in identifying its victims.

Confiscated bodies

One of the defining characteristics of the political violence of the Soviet period was that the bodies of its victims were never returned to their loved ones. The confiscation of bodies by the state was established from the outset as the standard procedure for the treatment of the corpses of detainees, following explicit instructions given in a circular issued by the supreme tribunal of the Pan-Russian Executive Committee, dated 14 October 1922.[18] This stipulated:

> The body of the shot individual must not be returned to anyone; it will be buried without any formality or ritual, dressed in the clothes worn

when shot, on the site of the execution of the sentence or in any other available place, *in such a way as to leave no trace of burial* or, alternatively, it will be sent to the mortuary for incineration.[19]

These provisions were progressively applied to all places where deaths occurred (prisons, camps, hospitals), irrespective of how prisoners died: not just for executions, but also for deaths caused by homicide, accidents or illness. It was therefore the Soviet state, and more specifically the various administrative departments of the camps placed under the direct and sole authority of the state security organs (the GPU, NKVD or KGB, according to the period in question) which had the job of dealing with prisoners' bodies and systematically ensuring that they would 'leave no trace'.

This explicitly stated desire on the part of the state not to hand back bodies may be seen to fit in a number of ways into the logic of a corrective re-education of 'deviant' minds by means of deportation and forced labour. For the only prisoners who could leave the gulag and return to normal Soviet life were those who had been 'brought into line' through work. The corpses of those who had failed to do so were thus quite logically and unceremoniously disposed of by the state through burial, immersion in water, cremation, or simply being abandoned in remote areas.

Burial, immersion in water, incineration, abandonment

Several techniques were thus used to dispose of the bodies of dead detainees 'in such a way as to leave no trace'. Individual burial was rare, tending to be used in networks of camps that had functioned for a sufficiently long period for their sites to have become permanent. In such cases, one finds funerary mounds, usually containing unmarked graves, but sometimes bearing the dead prisoner's number engraved on a piece of metal (taken from a tin can), or on a wooden stake.[20]

Mass burial was the method most frequently used. To this end, each administrative unit of the gulag system (Ourallag, Dmitlag, Volgolag, etc.) had gravedigging brigades composed of detainees assigned exclusively to logistical tasks relating to burial. The burial pits were dug directly on land administered by the state security services, in areas near to the sites of detention. The frequency at which they were dug was dependent on the rate of mortality in the camp, which could vary greatly.[21]

These mass graves were more often than not dug by hand, as attested by Dimitri Vassilievitch Ostroumov.[22] Born in Moscow in 1924, he was arrested in Leningrad in August 1942 and imprisoned there until February 1943. Sentenced to ten years' forced labour, he was initially placed in the Volgolag at Uglitch, then transferred to the Volgolag at Rybinsk, where he would remain until 1948, before being transferred to Norilsk, where he spent the rest of his sentence. While mainly given general work duties on the Rybinsk site, such as tree-felling and log-cutting, the young man was also assigned to the *Mogilŝiki* (gravediggers') brigade. He describes having thus participated in the daily digging of graves which could contain twenty to thirty corpses, situated on the outskirts of one of the civilian cemeteries of Rybinsk. However, these pits were occasionally dug using dynamite or ammonium nitrate in camps situated in polar or arctic regions, a practice which even gave rise to a specific term, *ammonalniki*, which denoted these pits dug in the permafrost using explosives, into which the corpses of prisoners were thrown once winter was over.[23]

Immersion was also used at times in zones where, in winter, the ground was frozen too hard to be dug. The bodies of detainees were thus thrown into streams, rivers, lakes or the sea through holes hacked into the ice, as documented by the camp guard Danzig Baldaev in his sketchbooks.[24]

Repeated references have also been made to corpses being simply abandoned. Prisoners could die outside the camp perimeter, either during routine movements (their daily work often involved long and arduous journeys) or during transfers from one establishment to another (life in the camps was punctuated by frequent transfers of prisoners, on foot or by train). The organization of the vast Soviet camp network was not infallible, and there were times when bodies were simply left where they had fallen. One of the most striking examples of this practice is documented by the historian Nicolas Werth in his study of the Island of Nazino, nicknamed the 'Island of Death' or 'Cannibal Island'.[25]

In what constituted something of an exception to the rule, however, detainees' bodies were cremated in Moscow at the newly opened Donskoï cemetery, where the crematorium, which began operating in 1927 (and continued up to 1970), was used from 1935 onwards to incinerate some of the victims of Stalin's purges. The rate varied: while 'only' 107 bodies were clandestinely cremated in 1937, the bodies of all the people executed in Moscow in 1940 were cremated on this site.[26] The crematorium at the new Donskoï cemetery in which these cremations were carried out was removed in 1970, and the church which had housed it was restored and reinstated as a place of worship. However, several commemorative plaques left by delegations from various countries (including Japan, Germany, Poland and Korea) act as reminders that the Soviet capital was the scene not only of mass murders, but also of mass cremations, well before the ovens of the Nazi camps.

The vast majority of corpses from the gulags, however, remain buried in the vicinity of the camps. And so, given that the camps were for the most part situated in the vicinity of urban conglomerations, the map of the gulags precisely matches the map of the population of the Soviet Union. Yet in spite of the proximity between the Soviet population, the camps and their mass graves, there has never been a systematic policy of locating burial sites (whether at local, regional or federal level), and no official inventory of mass graves has ever been drawn up. While the map of the camps has now been established,[27] the map of the mass graves of the gulags has yet to be drawn.

The return of human remains

The facts, though, stubbornly refuse to go away, and it is impossible to ignore the skeletons, hidden away for so long, that are now reappearing.

The reappearance of human remains can occur by chance due to a variety of factors, whether climatic (forest fires, floods, drought) or geological (landslides, soil erosion) in nature; it can also be the result of building works such as road widening, the construction of new buildings, or excavation beneath existing buildings to create car parks. Accidental and unexpected discoveries are just as likely to occur out in the countryside as they are on the outskirts of urban areas or in the middle of cities.

Thus, on 4 October 2007, workers on a construction site beneath an old apartment building in the centre of Moscow which was to be converted into a shopping centre discovered the remains of thirty-four bodies and a rusty pistol.[28] The obvious age of the skeletons and the bullet impacts visible on the skulls, indicating that they had been shot at point-blank range, along with the fact that the building was just opposite the infamous 'Rasstrelny Dom',[29] led the local police to presume that the remains were probably those of victims of the Great Purges of 1937–38. The spokesman for the regional coroner's office, however, opined that they might have 'died as a result of illness … during the Tsarist era'. The official report on the cause of death, which should have been released at the end of the inquest, has yet to be made public. In June 2010, meanwhile, a mass grave containing 500 skeletons (3.5 tonnes of bones in total) was discovered by workers building a road on the outskirts of Vladivostok.[30]

However, human remains can also reappear as a result of intentional excavations carried out to this end by various actors motivated by a dual desire both to bring the long-hidden dead to light and to give victims a proper reburial. Those who are attempting to locate sites of clandestine burial may be lone individuals (often interested in local history) whose motivations are frequently linked to very particular contexts of strong personal significance. Occasionally, Russian or sometimes even foreign institutions (as in the case of the Katyn massacre, in which various Polish institutions were involved) conduct searches. The Orthodox Church has thus been actively involved in the exhumations carried out on the site at Butovo in the Moscow suburbs, where mass graves were thought to contain the bodies of priests and monks, in order to identify these bodies and see to their reburial.[31] Some NGOs have also organized research expeditions along the same lines as the ethnographic and archaeological expeditions carried out in the nineteenth century by scientists and folklorists. Viatcheslav Bitioutskij, the regional organizer in Voronezh for the NGO Memorial has for more than twenty years (following the discovery in September 1989 of a first mass grave) been conducting a slow and painstaking investigation of the clandestine burials carried out in forested areas near Voronezh. This search has already led to the discovery of fifty-three pits containing the remains of 2,361 individuals, who have all subsequently been given a religious burial. Out of these, it has been possible to identify only a single group of forty-eight victims, and this was due to a stroke of luck: one of the victims had his arrest warrant in his pocket.[32]

The problem of identifying these bodies is the main stumbling block encountered by all procedures of exhumation (and reburial) in Russia, for while the archives of the state security organs meticulously document the details of the trial and sentencing process, they say absolutely nothing about the locations and techniques used to dispose of the bodies of executed prisoners (burial, cremation, immersion in water, abandonment). Although exhumations frequently do provide indications as to the historical context of their deaths, allowing a date to be assigned to the latter, the skeletons are rarely identified.

The treatment of human remains following their exhumation and the legal status assigned to them as individuals pose a new set of legal and political problems of a particularly thorny nature. It is by no means rare, then, for remains from gulag mass graves to be reburied outside of any legal framework, the coroner in question having either refused to open an inquest (thus avoiding having to make a decision regarding the legal status of the bones, which might place the responsibility for dealing with them on the state) or ruled that the human remains which have been discovered are archaeological artefacts without commercial value, and hence without national historical value, thereby absolving the state of any responsibility for them and allowing those who found them to do with them as they please. The reappearance of human remains several decades after the disappearance, then, poses Russian society with a series of complex and entirely new questions.

The status and social functions of human remains

These reappearances thus have a retrospective effect, forcing society to look back upon the long years during which it had lived alongside these skeletons strewn across its territory. It is therefore apposite in this context to examine the symbolic and social mechanisms which have legitimized such a long presence–absence of human remains on such a massive scale, and have made it possible to draw a veil of silence over this lengthy period spent in the company of countless mass graves. In this respect, whole sections of the social history of the USSR have yet to be written. An examination of this geography of shadows, this geography of the implicit (with all its whispered knowledge, its rumours), which was maintained over many decades and is now resurfacing due to a change in the political situation that also corresponds to a generational shift, surely constitutes one of the most promising avenues for future research in this area. In an academic context, a *true* sociology of denial, which Stanley Cohen has started to explore, stands to gain much from close attention to the ways in which multiple avoidance strategies, in particular those of a linguistic nature, have been deployed by, and subsequently become engrained within, Russian society.[33]

Indeed, the context of these reappearances corresponds in a number of ways to a return of the repressed. Following on from the work begun by Cara Krmpotich, Joost Fontein and John Harries on the agency of bones, in a very real sense, to become social actors, and in the light of what may be seen in Russia, it is necessary to consider not only what the return of human remains reveals to Russian society about its own past, but also which parts of the structures erected to maintain a consensus of silence around the presence of mass graves are imperilled by the discovery of those graves and their contents.[34]

Looking forward from these reappearances, meanwhile, it is equally important to study the agendas behind, on the one hand, the negotiations over the legal status of human remains (and consequently their ultimate fate) and, on the other, the actual practices of reburial. For the extremely prominent position that religious elements are now coming to occupy (both in the rituals being performed and in the memorials being erected), along with political and ideological interests (with the progressive growth of nationalist agendas in many territories born out of the disintegration of the USSR), forces us to consider, following on from the pioneering work by Katherine Verdery, the political and religious life of human remains, and to embark upon a true social anthropology of the practices of reburial in post-Soviet spaces.[35]

What do these bones represent?

Yet the return of the dead brings with it a set of radical methodological and epistemological questions for those studying post-Soviet societies.

If indeed we wish to pursue an analysis of this 'dark side of modernity' (*'face obscure de la modernité'*), to use Jackie Assayag's expression (2007), how can we 'come to an understanding' (*'faire avec'*) and deal with secrecy?[36] How can we distinguish between what has been known but silenced, or simply believed without ever having been seen, and how can we delimit the nebulous role of the collective imagination? On the ground, the richness and highly 'talkative' nature of archives form a counterpoint to the elisions, euphemisms, allusions and metaphors which characterize the testimony of survivors and neighbours of the camps alike, greatly complicating the task of the ethnographer when it comes to exploring a phenomenon of denial on such a scale.

Moreover, is the observational distance so prized by anthropologists still tenable when observing social configurations that are so deeply marked by extreme violence? In distancing ourselves do we not run the risk of remaining on the margins, of missing the true meaning of social behaviours? On a deeper level, how much importance should be attached to 'axiological neutrality', that founding principle of investigative work, when faced with the disgust, the fear or the incredulity which sometimes seize the researcher confronted with the material traces of the destruction of bodies? And how do we force ourselves to think the unthinkable, given that the logical and social frameworks which made the production of death on such a scale possible seem to escape any articulations of ordinary reasoning?

As regards the question of ethics, how do we avoid voyeurism and provide an intelligible account of the facts without sliding into obscenity? And, insofar as the victims are survived by executioners as well as witnesses (whose potential collaborative role in the violence is always far from clear at first), and given that the ethical principles of ethnographic investigation demand that we 'do not prejudice' our interviewees, how can we record the words of killers and of their potential accomplices? Finally, what ought to be the relationship between the researcher and human remains when the status bestowed upon these by the society under study is that of 'archaeological artefacts without commercial value', or even of simple refuse? Any researcher who carries out a real exploration of a field such as that of the traces left by practices of extreme violence, and in particular that of the social uses of human remains, can only hope to arrive at a series of subtle compromises, always unstable and always unsatisfactory, and often marked by half-retractions and false victories.

However, insofar as anthropology gives equal weight to what is left unsaid as to what is explicitly stated, the discipline is indeed able to shed light upon the densest and sometimes most illegible elements that acts and words may conceal within themselves. It thus allows us to establish a documented inventory of the present state of a society. The true challenge facing any anthropologist who really seeks to understand these mass crimes and reconstitute the long biography of their mass graves, as a witness to the witnesses of violence, confronted like them with the confusion or illegibility of traces, is that of accepting to work with tenuous clues and faltering trails. For this is the only way to establish a template for a true social symptomatology, which constitutes the only hope we have of exerting a truly beneficial influence on the discourse of legal experts and historians.

Practices of concealment and their effects

The application of these practices of concealment to the evidence of the gulag in turn poses the anthropologist, as well as the historian and the legal specialist, with a set of questions that are essential to understanding the social effects of extreme violence. However, in order to pursue this line of investigation further, it is necessary to clarify certain key points.

Firstly, as the case of the USSR clearly demonstrates, one of the principal social effects of the confiscation of bodies is to maintain the societies in question in a state of deferred mourning,[37] and this mourning can be deferred for a very long time indeed. For it is still practically impossible for the descendants of the 2 million who died in the gulags (some of whom perished in the 1930s) to know the date of the deaths of their loved ones, the conditions under which these occurred or the place of their burial, despite the fact that they died inside a state institution. The victims of this mass violence are in this respect comparable to the 'disappeared' of the Latin American dictatorships. It is also important to remember that the key feature of the crime of disappearance (characterized by the absence of a body), as opposed to that of homicide (where the corpse is the first piece of evidence pointing to the crime), is that it continues for as long as the victim remains undiscovered. On a purely legal level, then, mass violence which is accompanied by the confiscation, concealment or destruction of bodies must be considered as being distinct from mass murders committed without confiscation, and treated as a specific category of violence perpetrated over an extended period.

This first set of points shows the need for a more sustained investigation of the specific features and the wider implications of these practices of concealment in comparison with radically different practices such as the abandonment or indeed the intentional display of corpses. This is where the importance of a comparative analysis of the production of violence becomes clear.

By comparing the Soviet case with other practices of destruction or concealment, as applied, for example, in the context of the Holocaust through the use of specially designed cremation ovens,[38] under the Uruguayan dictatorship with the implementation of 'Operation Carrot',[39] or in the former Yugoslavia with the widespread use of secondary or tertiary burials,[40] it is possible to see that wherever the practice of confiscation of bodies by the state occurs, it is accompanied by the mobilization – or indeed the creation – of technological devices or practices which are specifically designed to facilitate the hiding of bodies, and which are distinct from techniques of killing.

This link between mass violence and technological innovation emerges within a historical context, that of the twentieth century, which was particularly marked by the growing complexity of devices used (going, for example, from using spades to using bulldozers to dig burial pits) and by the importance of transfers of technology. It should be noted, for example, that the same German firm, Topf & Söhne, which in 1926 designed the crematory ovens that would allow the Soviet state to carry out the clandestine incineration of the victims of the purges would, at the beginning of the 1940s, design crematory ovens able to function day and night and which were installed most notoriously at Auschwitz-Birkenau.

The circulation of techniques and knowledge is thus revealed as being at the heart of practices of the mass destruction of bodies, not merely at the stage of killing, but also at the subsequent, additional stages of the confiscation of bodies and the concealment of traces. These are all questions that have yet to be studied in detail in order to measure their true effects and social implications.

Notes

1 R. Hertz, 'Contribution à une étude sur la représentation collective de la mort', *L'Année Sociologique*, 10 (1907), pp. 48–137.
2 C. Rigeade, *Les Sépultures de catastrophe: approche anthropologique des sites d'inhumations en relation avec des épidémies de peste, des massacres de population et des charniers militaires* (BAR International S1695, internal report, 2007), p. 129; M. Signoli, D. Chevé, P. Adalian, G. Boëtsch & O. Dutour, *La Peste: entre épidémies et sociétés* (Florence: Firenze University Press, 2007); M. Signoli, 'Archéo-anthropologie funéraire et épidémiologie', *Socio-anthropologie*, 22 (2008), at http://socio-anthropologie.revues.org/index1155.html (accessed 2 October 2012).
3 O. Dutour, 'Traces de vies disparues: l'anthropologue face aux charniers', *Socio-anthropologie*, 12 (2002), at http://socio-anthropologie.revues.org/index146.html (accessed 27 November 2013).
4 J. Assayag, 'La face obscure de la modernité', *L'Homme*, 170 (2004), pp. 232–43.
5 F. Ferrandiz, 'Exhuming the defeated: civil war mass grave in 21st century Spain', *American Ethnologist*, 40:1 (2013), pp. 38–54.
6 E. Claverie, 'Réapparaître. Retrouver les corps des personnes disparues pendant la guerre en Bosnie', *Raisons Politiques*, 41:1 (2011), pp. 13–31.

7 The acronym GULag (*Glavnoe Upravlenie Lagerei*: principal camp authority) initially designated the administrative authority which oversaw the ITL (Ispravitel'no-Trudovoj Lager), the 're-education through work' camps. The term came to be used metonymically to refer to the institution as a whole, covering all the spaces of the Soviet concentration camp system.
8 An exhaustive list of the camps which operated between 1923 and 1960, giving details of dates of operation, numbers of personnel and detainees and their activities, has been published in Russian: N. Ohotin & A. Roginski, *Sistema ispravitel'no-trudovyh lagerei v SSSR, 1923–1960* (Moscow: Zvenia, 1998).
9 The camps were referred to as ITLs (*Ispravitelno-trudovye lageria*): literally, 're-education through work' camps (sometimes translated as 'correction by work' camps).
10 A. Becker, 'Exterminations: le corps et les camps', in J. J. Courtine (ed.), *Histoire du corps. Volume 3: Les mutations du regard, le XXe siècle* (Paris: Le Seuil, 2006), pp. 321–39.
11 A. Kokurin, N. Petrov & V. Sostakovic, *Gulag Glavnoe Upravlenie Lagerei 1917–1960* (Moskva: Demokra, 2000).
12 O. Khlevniuk, *The History of the Gulag: From Collectivization to the Great Terror* (New Haven: Yale University Press, 2000).
13 The work of Alexander Solzhenitsyn contributed to the popularization of the image of the gulag as an archipelago of islands, just as much as it raised awareness of its real nature.
14 See the analyses by the geographer R. Brunet, 'Géographie du goulag', *L'Espace géographique*, 3 (1981), pp. 215–32, and the work of the 'Mapping the Gulag' research programme, led by Judith Pallot (Oxford University), at www.gulagmaps.org (accessed 26 November 2013).
15 For an analysis of the involvement of the gulag in the Soviet economy, see G. M. Ivanova (ed.), *Labor Camp Socialism: The Gulag in the Soviet Totalitarian System* (New York: M. E. Sharpe, 2000).
16 For a rapid overview of the debates surrounding the number of victims of the Soviet camps, see the appendix to Anne Applebaum, *Gulag a History of the Soviet Camps* (London: Penguin Books, 2003), pp. 515–22.
17 See chapter 10, 'Le phénomène concentrationnaire soviétique au XXe siècle', of N. Werth, *La Terreur et le désarroi: Staline et son système* (Paris: Perrin, 2007), pp. 199–221, in particular the table on p. 221.
18 The administrative ancestor of the Supreme Soviet of the USSR, the Pan-Russian Executive Committee (PREC) constituted the highest executive institution of the state.
19 PREC circular of 14 October 1922 as quoted in E. Jemkova, 'Les répressions staliniennes à Moscou et les lieux d'inhumation de masse', in É. Anstett & L. Jurgenson (eds), *Le Goulag en héritage: pour une anthropologie de la trace* (Paris: Pétra, 2009), p. 115. Emphasis added.
20 See the photographs taken by Ivan Panikarov to accompany his article 'Le chemin s'arrête-t-il là?', in Anstett & Jurgenson, *Le Goulag en héritage*, pp. 131–41.

21 Memorial, a non-governmental organization (NGO), has begun drawing up an inventory of the mass graves sited on the territory of the former USSR. Its website, Gulagmuseum.org, contains a section devoted specifically to burial sites entitled 'Nekropoli', but, as of November 2013, it had only 522 entries. See http://gulagmuseum.org/search.do?objectTypeName=necropolis&page=1&language=1 (accessed 24 November 2013).
22 Memorial archives, Fond 1, delo 3449, opis 1.
23 For further explanation of gulag vocabulary, see J. Rossi, *Le Manuel du goulag* (Paris: Le Cherche Midi, 1997).
24 D. Baldaev, *Drawings from the Gulag* (London: Fuel, 2010). See the drawings on p. 89 and following, in particular that on p. 95.
25 N. Werth, *L'Île aux cannibales: 1933, une déportation-abandon en Sibérie* (Paris: Perrin, 2006).
26 The number of clandestine cremations carried out at the Donskoï cemetery was more than 1,500 (probably nearer 1,800) according to estimates based on the archives of the state security organs. See Jemkova, 'Les répressions staliniennes à Moscou', p. 123.
27 See the animated maps created by the group of geographers led by Judith Pallot at www.gulagmaps.org/maps (accessed May 2014).
28 See the report by the news agency Reuters dated 4 October 2007 and circulated by various media outlets, including *The Guardian* – see www.guardian.co.uk/world/2007/oct/05/russia.international (accessed 25 November 2013).
29 Referred to as the 'House of Execution', the building at 23 Nikolskaya Street housed the Military College of the Supreme Tribunal of the USSR, which, in Moscow alone, sentenced more than 40,000 people to capital punishment. It is also significant that the building site at which the bodies were found was situated just a few blocks away from the Lubyanka, the former headquarters of the NKVD (Narodnyy Komissariat Vnutrennikh Del, the People's Commissariat for Internal Affairs, responsible for the state security services and secret police), and current headquarters of the FSB (Federal'naya sluzhba bezopasnosti Rossiyskoy Federatsii, Federal Security Service of the Russian Federation, the direct successor to the USSR's Committee of State Security, or KGB).
30 See www.themoscowtimes.com/news/article/stalin-era-grave-yields-tons-of-bones/408048.html (accessed May 2014).
31 See the article by K. Rousselet, 'Butovo: la création d'un lieu de pèlerinages sur une terre de massacres', *Politix*, 20 (2007), p. 55–78. For a bibliography of historical research on this site, see the article by F.-X. Nérard for the online *Encyclopaedia of Mass Violence* entitled 'The Butovo shooting range', at www.massviolence.org/The-Butovo-Shooting-Range?artpage=6 (accessed May 2014).
32 See V. Bitioutskij, 'Tragiceskij pamiatnik bolchogo terrora v Voroneje', *30' Oktiabria*, 103 (2011), pp. 8–9.
33 S. Cohen, *State of Denial: Knowing About Atrocities and Suffering* (Cambridge: Polity Press, 2001).

34 C. Krmpotich, J. Fontein & J. Harries, 'The substance of bones: the emotive materiality and affective presence of human remains', *Journal of Material Culture*, 15:4 (2010), pp. 371–84.
35 K. Verdery, *Political Lives of Dead Bodies: Reburial and Post-socialist Change* (New York: Columbia University Press, 1999).
36 J. Assayag, 'Le spectre des génocides', *Gradhiva*, 5 (2007), pp. 6–25, http://gradhiva.revues.org/658 (accessed 16 April 2013).
37 É. Anstett, 'Mémoire des répressions politiques en Russie postsoviétique: le cas du Goulag' (17 July 2011), *Online Encyclopedia of Mass Violence*, at www.massviolence.org/Memoire-des-repressions-politiques-en-Russie-postsovietique (accessed 5 October 2012).
38 R. J. van Pelt, *The Case for Auschwitz: Evidence from the Irving Trial* (Bloomington: Indiana University Press, 2002).
39 J. Lopez Mazz, 'Historias desaparecidas y re aparecidas: el caso de Uruguay', in A. Zaranquin, M. Salerno & C. Perosino (eds), *Historias desaparecidas: arqueología, memoria y violencia política* (Cordoba: Brujas, 2012), pp. 45–60.
40 Claverie, 'Réapparaître'.

Bibliography

Anstett, É., 'Mémoire des répressions politiques en Russie postsoviétique: le cas du Goulag' (17 July 2011), in *Online Encyclopedia of Mass Violence*, at www.massviolence.org/Memoire-des-repressions-politiques-en-Russie-postsovietique

Anstett, É. & L. Jurgenson (eds), *Le Goulag en héritage: pour une anthropologie de la trace* (Paris: Pétra, 2009), from the series 'Sociétés et cultures postsoviétiques en mouvement', directed by M. Laruelle and V. Symaniec

Applebaum, A., *Gulag a History of the Soviet Camps* (London: Penguin Books, 2003)

Assayag, J., 'La face obscure de la modernité', *L'Homme*, 170 (2004), pp. 232–43

Assayag, J., 'Le spectre des génocides', *Gradhiva*, 5 (2007), pp. 6–25, http://gradhiva.revues.org/658

Baldaev, D., *Drawings from the Goulag* (London: Fuel, 2010)

Becker, A., 'Exterminations: le corps et les camps', in J. J. Courtine (ed.), *Histoire du corps. Volume 3: Les mutations du regard, le XXe siècle* (Paris: Le Seuil, 2006), pp. 321–39

Bitioutskij, V., 'Tragiceskij pamiatnik bolchogo terrora v Voroneje', *30' Oktiabria*, 103 (2011), pp. 8–9

Brunet, R., 'Géographie du goulag', *L'Espace géographique*, 3 (1981), pp. 215–32

Claverie, E., 'Réapparaître. Retrouver les corps des personnes disparues pendant la guerre en Bosnie', *Raisons Politiques*, 41:1 (2011), pp. 13–31

Cohen, S., *State of Denial: Knowing About Atrocities and Suffering* (Cambridge: Polity Press, 2001)

Dutour, O., 'Traces de vies disparues: l'anthropologue face aux charniers', *Socio-anthropologie*, 12 (2002), at http://socio-anthropologie.revues.org/index146.html

Ferrandiz, F., 'Exhuming the defeated: civil war mass grave in 21st century Spain', *American Ethnologist*, 40:1 (2013), pp. 38–54

Héritier, F., *De la violence II* (Paris: Odile Jacob, 1999)

Hertz, R., 'Contribution à une étude sur la représentation collective de la mort', *L'Année Sociologique*, 10 (1907), pp. 48–137

Ivanova, G. M. (ed.), *Labor Camp Socialism: The Gulag in the Soviet Totalitarian System* (New York: M. E. Sharpe, 2000)

Jemkova, E., 'Les répressions staliniennes à Moscou et les lieux d'inhumation de masse', in É. Anstett & L. Jurgenson (eds), *Le Goulag en héritage: pour une anthropologie de la trace* (Paris: Pétra, 2009), pp. 115–29

Khlevniuk, O., *The History of the Gulag: From Collectivization to the Great Terror* (New Haven: Yale University Press, 2000)

Kokurin, A., N. Petrov & V. Sostakovic, *Gulag Glavnoe Upravlenie Lagerei 1917–1960* (Moskva: Demokra, 2000)

Krmpotich, C., J. Fontein & J. Harries, 'The substance of bones: the emotive materiality and affective presence of human remains', *Journal of Material Culture*, 15:4 (2010), pp. 371–84

Lopez Mazz, J., 'Historias desaparecidas y re aparecidas: el caso de Uruguay', in A. Zaranquin, M. Salerno & C. Perosino (eds), *Historias desaparecidas: arqueología, memoria y violencia política* (Cordoba: Brujas, 2012), pp. 45–60

Naepels, M., 'Quatre questions sur la violence', *L'Homme*, 177–8 (2006), pp. 487–95

Ohotin, N. & A. Roginski, *Sistema ispravitel'no-trudovyh lagerei v SSSR, 1923–1960* (Moscow: Zvenia, 1998)

Panikarov, I., 'Le chemin s'arrête-t-il là?', in E. Anstett & L. Jurgenson (eds), *Le Goulag en héritage: pour une anthropologie de la trace* (Paris: Pétra, 2009), pp. 131–41

Platt, T., *Grave Matters: Excavating California's Buried Past* (Berkeley: Heyday, 2011)

Rigeade, C., *Les Sépultures de catastrophe: approche anthropologique des sites d'inhumations en relation avec des épidémies de peste, des massacres de population et des charniers militaires* (BAR International S1695, internal report, 2007)

Rossi, J., *Le Manuel du goulag* (Paris: Le Cherche Midi, 1997)

Rousselet, K., 'Butovo: la création d'un lieu de pèlerinages sur une terre de massacres', *Politix*, 20 (2007), pp. 55–78

Signoli, M., 'Archéo-anthropologie funéraire et épidémiologie', *Socio-anthropologie*, 22 (2008), published 14 October 2009, at http://socio-anthropologie.revues.org/index1155.html

Signoli, M., D. Chevé, P. Adalian, G. Boëtsch & O. Dutour, *La Peste: entre épidémies et sociétés* (Florence: Firenze University Press, 2007)

Van Pelt, R. J., *The Case for Auschwitz: Evidence from the Irving Trial* (Bloomington: Indiana University Press, 2002)

Verdery, K., *Political Lives of Dead Bodies: Reburial and Post-socialist Change* (New York: Columbia University Press, 1999)

Werth, N., 'Un état contre son peuple: violences, répressions, terreurs en URSS de 1917 à 1953', in S. Courtois (ed.), *Le Livre noir du communisme* (Paris: Robert Laffont, 1998), pp. 41–295

Werth, N., *L'Île aux cannibales: 1933, une déportation-abandon en Sibérie* (Paris: Perrin, 2006)

Werth, N., *La Terreur et le désarroi: Staline et son système* (Paris: Perrin, 2007)

Index

abduction of children 49
abjection, theory of 26
Adenauer, Konrad 135
Agamben, Giorgio 12, 16, 18
Agnew, Robert S. 90
Akayesu case 59–60, 67–8
Alfonsín, Raúl 47
Allach 136
American Anthropological
 Association 34
American Association of Physical
 Anthropologists 33–4
amnesties 47
Ang Choulean 155
Antelme, Robert 72
anthropometry 83
Argentina 44–8, 94–6, 168
 Supreme Court 50
Arusha Accords (1993) 165
Assayag, Jackie 190
Auschwitz 64, 107, 131, 135, 161, 167, 193
axiological neutrality 191
Ayen, Duchess of 140

Bagosora, Théoneste 165
Baldaev, Danzig 186
Bandura, Albert 90
Bataille, G. 25, 28
battlefields 27
Bauman, Zygmunt 166
Bemba Gombo case 61
Benjamin, Walter 44
Bergen-Belsen 136, 139
Bignone, Reynaldo 47
biodisciplinary power 16–18
biographic interview technique 154
biopolitics 12–25, 31, 34–5
 definitions of 14–15
 of genocide 19, 24
 historicist 15, 17–18, 21–2, 31
 naturalist 14–15, 17, 25
 ontologist 16–18, 20, 23, 31
 organistic 34
 politicist 15, 17
Bitioutskij, Viatcheslav 188
Blobel, Paul 119–20
bodies, dead
 abandonment of 186, 192
 confiscation by the state 184–5, 192–3
 as didactic objects 167–8
 disappearance of 45–6, 51
 and the escalation of violence 25–6
 as evidence 22, 62–71, 151, 153
 identification of 136–40
 judicial interest in 57–60

large concentrations of 32–3
legal status of 189–90
managed disposal of 32
materiality and physical
  presence of 27–32, 35
reappearance of 187–90
reasons for destruction of 66–7, 72
social treatment of 181–2
Bollas, Christopher 91
'bones-as-evidence' 151, 153
Bosanska Krupa 118
Breton, Stéphane 146
Brown, Peter 29
burial pits 154
Burundi 166–7
bystander effects 92

Cambodia 147–57
camps, death in 64, 112–15, 120, 131–2, 182–7
carabinieri 116
'catastrophe burial' concept 181
caves, disposal of bodies in 110–13, 116
Chandler, David 148
Choeung Ek 152
Christianity 29–30, 170–1
  see also Orthodox Church; Roman Catholic Church
Claverie, Elisabeth 182
'closure' 96–7
Cohen, Stanley 92, 189
Cold War 86, 151
Colombia 167–8
concealment of bodies 192–3
concentration camps see camps, death in
Copes, Heith 89
corpses see bodies, dead
'Corpses of Mass Violence and Genocide' research programme 3–6
correlationism 22–4
Cox, Simon 68
cremation 154, 186–7
crimes against humanity 57–9, 62
  definition of 57–8
criminology
  biological 84
  engagement with corpses 83–7

Croatia 106–20
'cultures of terror' 161, 167–8

Darfur 92
death
  change in the meaning of 30–1
  fear of 25
death marches 132, 135
dehumanization 64
demonstrative violence 117–19
denial strategies 89–95
Desforges, Alison 68
dignity, human 57, 61–2
disappearance and 'the disappeared' 44–50, 60, 192
disciplinary power 15–16, 22
DNA tests 49–50
Donauwörth 136
Donskoï cemetery 186–7
Douglas, Merry 25

Eichmann, Adolf 85
Einsatzgruppen 130
Elias, Norbert 83
enslavement 59–60
epidemics 32
Esposito, Roberto 16, 18–19
ethics committees 99
ethnographic research 99, 147, 170, 190–1
Euro-centrism 20
exposure of bodies 171–2

Ferrandiz, Francisco 182
First World War 19–20, 129–30
foibe 112
Fontein, Joost 25–6, 30, 167–8, 189–90
forensic anthropology 32–4
Foucault, Michel 4–5, 15–16, 18, 21–3, 29–31
François-Poncet, André 134
Freud, Sigmund 88–9

Garland, David 87
genocide 16–23, 35, 56, 65–71, 92–3, 161, 167, 169
  colonial 20
  definition of 62–3
genocide studies 2–3, 20
genocide tourism 153

Gerlach, Christian 21, 24, 27
Glueck, Sheldon 84
Gorbachev, Mikhail 183
gulag system 182–4, 187, 192
gushaka ishyamba 171
gypsies, mass murder of 114

Habyarimana, Juvénal 164–5
Hagan, John 86, 92–3, 99
Hamitic hypothesis 169, 172
Hardt, Michel 16–17
Harman, Graham 26
Harries, John 189–90
Heidegger, Martin 22–3
Hertz, Robert 181
Hilsum, Lindsey 68
Hitler, Adolf 107
Holocaust, the 19–20, 85, 97, 130, 192
human remains *see* bodies, dead
human rights 47–51
Hutu 162–7

Ieng Sary 152
Inter-American Commission on Human Rights 48
Inter-American Court of Human Rights 47
International Commission on Missing Persons (ICMP) 96
International Convention for the Protection of All Persons from Enforced Disappearance 48
International Criminal Court (ICC) 59–61, 63, 67
  see also Rome Statute
international criminal law 57
International Criminal Tribunal for Rwanda (ICTR) 56–9, 62, 67–8, 170
International Criminal Tribunal for the former Yugoslavia (ICTY) 56–60, 67–71, 99

Jadovno 113
Jasenovac 114–15, 120

Kafka, Franz 64–5, 166
Kagame, Aléxis 171
Kajelijeli case 62

Kalfa, Ariane 64
Kambanda, Jean 165
Kant, Immanuel 22
Karamira, Frodauld 165
Katanga and Ngudjolo Chui case 60
Katyn massacre 188
Kayibanda, Grégoire 163–4
Keane, Fergal 170
Khleang Mueng 148–9, 155
Khmer Rouge 147–57
Kigali 170
'killing fields' 114
Kirchner, Nestor 47
Kochendorf 137
Koenig, General 132
Kotorani 109
Kristeva, Julia 25–6, 28
Krmpotich, Cara 189–90
Krstić case 69
Kukunjevac 117
Kunarac case 60

Lebensphilosophie 17, 28–9
Lefeuvre-Déotte, M. 45
Lemke, Thomas 18
Levi, Primo 166
Levinas, Emmanuel 72
Lombroso, Cesare 83
Luhmann, Niklas 15

Malkki, Lisa 166
Maruna, Shadd 89, 91, 95–6
mass violence
  academic studies of 2–3
  biopolitical interpretation of 18–21
  examples of 1–2
Matza, David 89–90, 92
Mbembe, Achille 19
McDoom, Omar 170
Meillassoux, Quentin 22
Mendès-France, Pierre 135
Menem, Carlos 47
Merleau-Ponty, M. 23
Mironko, Charles 170
Mitterand, François 164
moral arousal management 82–3, 88–99
  integrative potential of 93–7
  methodological and ethical issues 97–9

moral–emotional 'work' of crime 81–3, 87–8, 100
Morrison, Wayne 87
Moscow 186–7
Moses, Dirk A. 19
mourning, deferred 192
Mugesera, Léon 169
Mussolini, Benito 107

nation-states 17
Nazi regime 19–21, 64, 131, 184
  see also Einsatzgruppen; SS; Wehrmacht
Nazino Island 186
Ndadaye, Melchior 165
Negri, Antonio 16–17
Neitzel, Sonke 98
'neutralization' of moral problems 89–93
Nsengiyaremye, Dismas 164

oral history 22
Orthodox Church 188
Ostroumov, Dimitri Vassilievitch 186
ovens, crematory 193

Pag 113
Palančište 116–17
paramilitary conflicts 109
persecution, crime of 59
Piédelièvre, René 137
Piralian, Hélène 64–6
Plaza de Mayo, mothers of 45–6
Pol Pot 150, 152–3
power *see* biodisciplinary power; disciplinary power; sovereign power
privacy, right to 49–50
psychic distance 72

Quintyn, Conrad B. 34

racial classification 34
rape 60–1, 118–19
Ratisbonne 136–7
Reato, Ceferino 44–5
Reljevo 109
Renzaho, Tharcisse 170
repatriation of bodies 132–3, 136

rivers, disposal of corpses in 109–10, 114–15, 169
Robben, Antonius 168
Roman Catholic Church 171
Rome Statute 57–8, 88
Rousset, David 64
Rwanda 162–72

saints, cult of 29
Samrong Knong monastery 156
Sartre, Jean-Paul 25
Sauvagnargues, Jean 134
Schmitt, Carl 17
Scilingo, Adolfo 47
search missions 5, 131–4, 138–40
Second World War 20, 106–7, 130
Sémelin, Jacques 72–3
sexual slavery 59–60
sexual violence 61–2, 118–19
somatotyping 84
sovereign power 16, 18, 30
Soviet Union (USSR) 183–4, 190, 192
Srebrenica 69–71, 95, 161
SS (Schutz-Staffel) 72
Stepputat, Finn 25
sterilization, forced 58
Stone, Dan 20, 24, 27, 35
Sykes, Gresham 89–90

Taussig, Michael 167
Taylor, Anne-Christine 147
Taylor, Charles 28
Taylor, Christopher 166, 169
Topf & Söhne (company) 193
torture 58
transitional justice 82, 95, 99
truth, the, right to 48–51
tutelary spirits 155–6
Tutsi 162–6, 171–2

United Nations Commission on Human Rights 48, 50
United Nations Human Rights Council 48
Uribe, Maria Victoria 167
Uruguay 192
Ustaša militias 107–20

Vaihingen 136
Vallois, Henri-Victor 137

van't Spijker, Gerard 171
Verdery, Katherine 190
Verne, Jules 110
Versailles, Treaty of 134
Vidal, Claudine 170–1
Videla, Jorge 44–5
Vietnam and the Vietnam War 150–2
violence
   as a discursive practice 166
   participatory nature of 21–2
Voltaire 181

warlord regimes 108, 118
Wehrmacht, the 116–19
Welzer, Harald 98
Werth, Nicolas 186
Wörsdörfer, Rolf 112

Zachariah, Dr 68
Zimbabwe 26, 30, 168

EU authorised representative for GPSR:
Easy Access System Europe, Mustamäe tee 50,
10621 Tallinn, Estonia
gpsr.requests@easproject.com

www.ingramcontent.com/pod-product-compliance
Ingram Content Group UK Ltd.
Pitfield, Milton Keynes, MK11 3LW, UK
UKHW021841140426